Assessing Changing Food Consumption Patterns

Committee on Food Consumption Patterns

Food and Nutrition Board
National Research Council

NATIONAL ACADEMY PRESS
Washington, D.C. 1981

NOTICE The project that is the subject of this report was approved by the Governing Board of the National Research Council, whose members are drawn from the Councils of the National Academy of Sciences, the National Academy of Engineering, and the Institute of Medicine. The members of the Committee responsible for the report were chosen for their special competences and with regard for appropriate balance.

This report has been reviewed by a group other than the authors according to procedures approved by a Report Review Committee consisting of members of the National Academy of Sciences, the National Academy of Engineering, and the Institute of Medicine.

The National Research Council was established by the National Academy of Sciences in 1916 to associate the broad community of science and technology with the Academy's purposes of furthering knowledge and of advising the federal government. The Council operates in accordance with general policies determined by the Academy under the authority of its Congressional charter of 1863, which establishes the Academy as a private, nonprofit, self-governing membership corporation. The Council has become the principal operating agency of both the National Academy of Sciences and the National Academy of Engineering in the conduct of their services to the government, the public, and the scientific and engineering communities. It is administered jointly by both Academies and the Institute of Medicine. The National Academy of Engineering and the Institute of Medicine were established in 1964 and 1970, respectively, under the charter of the National Academy of Sciences.

The study summarized in this report was supported by Contract 223-77-2060 from the Food and Drug Administration, Public Health Service, Department of Health, Education and Welfare.

Library of Congress Cataloging in Publication Data

National Research Council (U.S.). Committee on
Food Consumption Patterns.
Assessing changing food consumption patterns.

Bibliography: p.
1. Nutrition surveys—United States. 2. Food
consumption—United States. I. Title.
TX360.U6N33 1981 641'.0973 81-9476
ISBN 0-309-03135-4 AACR2

Available from

NATIONAL ACADEMY PRESS
2101 Constitution Avenue, N.W.
Washington, D.C. 20418

Printed in the United States of America

COMMITTEE ON FOOD CONSUMPTION PATTERNS

ROBERT O. NESHEIM, The Quaker Oats Company, *Chairman*
I. J. ABRAMS, Market Research Corporation of America
HENRY BLACKBURN, University of Minnesota
DORIS H. CALLOWAY, University of California at Berkeley
HELEN A. GUTHRIE, The Pennsylvania State University
TIMOTHY M. HAMMONDS, Food Marketing Institute
GAIL G. HARRISON, University of Arizona
HAROLD B. HOUSER, Case Western Reserve University

NAS/NRC Staff

MARGARET R. STEWART
MYRTLE L. BROWN
KENNETH R. FULTON

Preface

The Food and Nutrition Board established a Steering Committee to undertake the reported study. Members of the Committee on Food Consumption Patterns were drawn from several disciplines, including nutrition, anthropology, statistics, food economics, and epidemiology. Persons familiar with survey methodology as used in the various government agencies, academic institutions, and the private sector were included. The Committee gathered information from a variety of sources and organized a series of workshops to draw on the skills and experience of a large number of individuals and organizations.

Although the system is intended to meet the special needs of the Food and Drug Administration, it should be relevant for use by other agencies and institutions engaged in monitoring food consumption and nutritional and health status. The system can be used to screen a representative sample of the U.S. population or adapted for use in more detailed studies of specific population groups. Although economic and other considerations may influence adoption of the proposed system, the Committee believes that the method is valid and that the information gathered thereby would be significantly more complete and useful than methods that are currently available.

The Committee wishes to express its appreciation to the participants in its three workshops. Their contributions of background papers and thoughtful discussion were essential to development of the system proposed in this report. These papers are attached to the report in Appendixes A, B, and C. Participants in the workshops are listed in Appendix D.

The Committee also wishes to recognize the important contributions of George H. Beaton in development of some of the basic concepts of the proposed system.

Contents

Introduction

The Food and Nutrition Board of the National Academy of Sciences under contract from the Food and Drug Administration (FDA) was charged to study the sources of data on food consumption and to suggest a system for integrating these data with data on nutrition and health status. The purposes of the study were to evaluate current means of determining food consumption patterns and nutritional status and to devise alternative methods for obtaining information on food consumption, food consumption patterns, and nutritional status.

FDA's interest in this subject is not unique. The White House Conference on Food, Nutrition and Health (1969) discussed the need for better surveillance data, and the General Accounting Office (1978) has detailed the need for improved food and nutrition information systems in the United States. Similarly, the Office of Science and Technology Policy (1977) and the Office of Technology Assessment (1978) have identified nutrition surveillance as an important priority. The Surgeon General's recent report, *Promoting Health, Preventing Disease: Objectives for the Nation* (Department of Health and Human Services, 1980), cites the need for a national nutrition surveillance system and for integration of various data sets to provide locally useful information for nutrition planning. While the need for appropriate systems of measuring food consumption and nutritional status is broadly recognized, such systems are relatively expensive and must be properly designed to provide appropriate information on a cost-effective basis.

Reliable data concerning food consumption of individuals are needed for various reasons. They are important for adequate assessment of the nutritional value of the U.S. food supply, for assessment of the intake of incidental contaminants and of currently approved and possible new food additives, and for development of food fortification policies and nutritional quality standards for food products.

Regulators of the safety and nutritional efficacy of the food supply are concerned with linkages between food consumption patterns* and health. Changes in the world's economy and changes in food costs and availability, including the introduction of new products, may have a marked effect on food consumption patterns of individuals and population groups. An ability to forecast the possible influences of these changes upon nutrient intake and on the population's health and productivity would allow formulation of sound policies and programs with respect to food fortification, consumer education, nutrition and food intervention, and the like. In the final analysis, the requirements for appropriate food consumption data relate to health promotion and prevention of adverse health responses in the population.

The primary uses for which FDA and other agencies may require data on food consumption patterns linked to nutrition and health are summarized in the following list. This summary, while not exhaustive, does illustrate those purposes the Committee considered while developing this report.

1. Nutritional Considerations
   - to identify foods that are the primary contributors of key nutrients in the diet for various groups
   - to identify size and nature of populations whose health is at risk due to inadequate or excessive consumption of a nutrient
   - to obtain more extensive and valid data on the potential relationships of food consumption patterns to nutritional and health status
   - to identify foods most appropriate for use in supplying specific nutrients in fortification programs for populations at risk
   - to measure the effectiveness of food fortification programs in reducing the size of the populations at risk
2. Toxicological Considerations
   - to identify the primary patterns of use of foods and food components in the diets of a population
   - to identify extreme or unusual patterns of intake of foods or food ingredients including additives
   - to identify size and nature of populations at risk from use of certain foods or food products
   - to determine amount and/or number of food items in which a food additive may be permitted

*"Food consumption patterns" as used in this document refer to combinations of foods that constitute an individual's usual dietary intake, which includes daily and longer cyclical variations.

- to determine the need to modify regulations in response to changes in food consumption
- to determine intake of incidental contaminants and food additives

3. Historical and/or Secular Trends
    - to evaluate the past history of food consumption patterns of populations, particularly as related to economic, technological, or other factors
    - to predict changes in food consumption patterns as they may be influenced by economic, technological, or other developments

Characteristics of a System for Measuring Food Consumption Patterns

The following characteristics are considered by the Committee to be essential to any system designed to measure food consumption patterns of individuals and population groups.

- The system must be based on statistically valid and practical sampling procedures of the population or identified target population groups. It should have sufficient flexibility to be adapted to widely different target population groups, not only on a demographic basis, but also on the basis of patterns of food use. The system may have a number of subparts.
- The system should provide for adequate description and characterization of the target population groups on which data are obtained.
- The validity and reliability of the data obtained must be sufficient to meet the requirements of the proposed end use of the data. Analysis needs must be identified early in the course of the study.
- The collection, analysis, and reporting of data must be sufficiently rapid to provide timely information. Thus the system must have an efficient data reduction system including coding and editing.
- The system should provide data on usual and extreme intake patterns, i.e., assess the variability of food intake within the population groups in relation to potential consequences on nutrition and health status.
- The system should be capable of detecting and predicting trends, through ongoing sampling and by retrospective analysis. The system should lend itself to reliable subsampling for obtaining interim or trend data on specific population groups.

- The system should be designed to meet the various data requirements of a broad variety of user groups
- The system must be cost effective—that is, the information obtained must be of sufficient value to justify the cost of obtaining it.

The issues of privacy and confidentiality of data must be addressed in any system that collects information on individuals. If health and economic data are to be linked with dietary information, the issue is particularly critical. Appropriate safeguards for ensuring protection of privacy must be built into the system design at every stage. Not only is this a basic ethical concern, but concern for privacy will directly affect both subjects' willingness to respond and the validity of responses given.

At the present time many agencies, institutions, and individuals are involved in studies to assess food consumption and nutritional and health status of individuals and population groups. However, lack of common sampling designs and sociodemographic data makes it difficult to integrate or properly evaluate data obtained from these different sources. Lack of standardized collection methods and internal quality control is often a limiting factor. In order to expand the use of collected data, strong consideration should be given to making original data from studies available to other investigators. The sharing of data may eliminate much duplication and result in more cost-effective use of available information.

Relating Food Consumption Data and Nutritional Status Data

The value of food consumption data in relation to public health is realized when the data are processed to yield estimates of nutrient intake and of exposure to food additives and contaminants. It is not possible to assess nutritional status from dietary data alone. It is possible, however, to provide an estimate of the prevalence of individuals within a population group with intakes below requirements, and, with current knowledge of human requirements, it is possible to assess the individual's probability of inadequate status based on intake of some (but not all) nutrients. It is also possible to consider the potential risk of excessive intake of nutrients and of natural or added food components, i.e., food ingredients and additives, if the association between level of intake and risk of toxicity is known.

Health status indicators believed to be associated with food or nutrient intake can be identified if current dietary data can be linked to existing health data. Through appropriate studies of the food consumption patterns of individuals in a group, it would then be feasible to predict the prevalence of individuals who may have increased risk to their health from a particular pattern of food or nutrient intake.

Environmental variables in addition to diet (such as endemic infectious disease or unusual stress) may increase the prevalence of nutritional inadequacy from that indicated by nutrient intake. In the United States, these other factors, with the possible exception of recurrent infections in children, probably do not generally contribute to variability of requirements, and therefore a valid estimate of risk can be generated by appropriate collection and analysis of dietary data.

The following discussion of an approach to the data collection system focuses primarily on application of the information to a prediction of nutritional status. The same system could be used for assessing toxicological risk and, with some modifications that will be discussed later, for relating food consumption to various aspects of health (growth, longevity, chronic diseases, etc.).

The linkage between dietary intake and nutritional status is portrayed in Figure 1. Interest is in the usual situation on a particular day. Thus, the data essential to this system are *usual* intake of food, *usual* composition of foods, *usual* bioavailability of nutrients, and *usual* nutrient requirement of the individual. There is no precise definition of the time span represented by "usual," but for purpose of discussion it may be taken as the average value persisting over a period of weeks rather than a day or two.

The statistical approach to analysis and to the prediction of the prevalence of individuals with usual intakes below their actual requirements has been identified and discussed by Lörstad (1971). It has been applied in a prediction of the effects of iron fortification on the prevalence of inadequate intakes among menstruating women (Swiss and Beaton, 1974) and in the identification of protein:energy ratios associated with predetermined prevalences of individuals having inadequate intakes (Beaton and Swiss, 1974). This statistical approach is based on the bivariate distribution of intakes and of requirements among individuals in the population. It is applicable to a dietary analysis system designed to monitor conditions in the United States.

Analyses based upon the bivariate distribution require knowledge of (1) the distribution of usual intakes (mean, variability), (2) the distribution of usual requirements (mean, variability), and (3) the correlation between intake and requirement among individuals (FAO/WHO, 1973). For many nutrients, requirements are at first-order approximations; and for most nutrients, but not energy, the correlation between intake and requirement appears to be very low and may be ignored provided that care is taken to express the data in a manner that avoids the effect of common variables such as body size, energy intake, etc. In the case of energy, intake and requirement of the individual are generally matched relatively closely, probably through physiologic regulatory mechanisms. Thus, a high correlation between intake and requirement would be expected. For various micronutrients, there is little or no reason to expect a correlation between intake and requirement unless both relate to a third variable. For example, thiamin intake is likely to relate to total energy intake and thiamin requirement is believed to be related to energy utilization. If intake and requirement are both expressed as milligrams per day, a spurious correlation may appear. This error can be avoided by expressing intake in a manner (such as mg/1,000 kcal), which controls for the confounding variable.

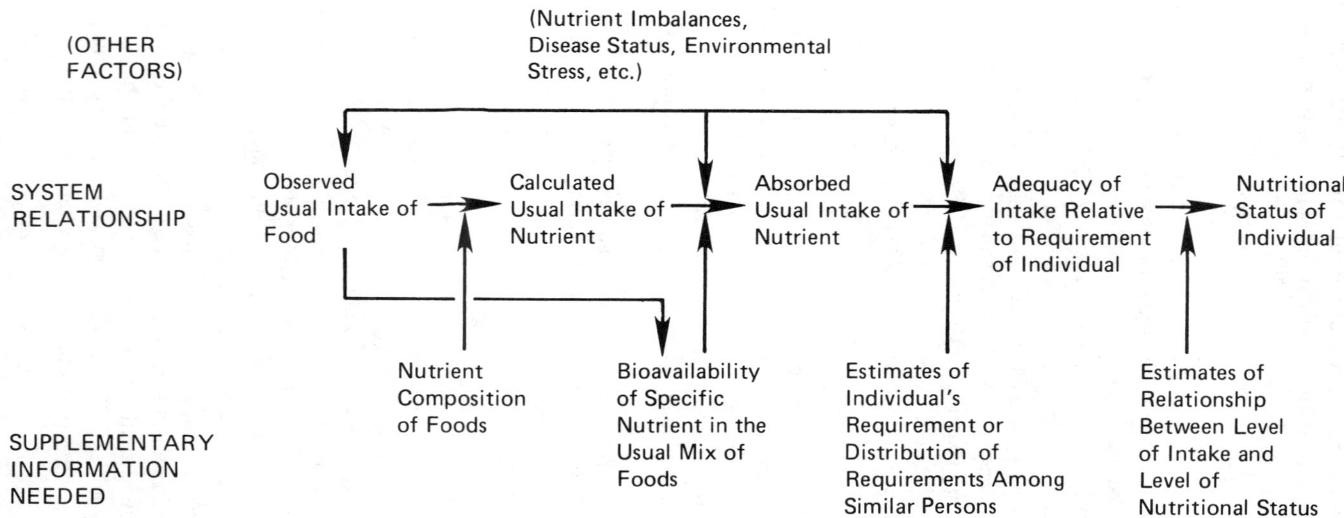

FIGURE 1 A system for analysis and interpretation of dietary data.

Attention must focus on the need for information about the distribution of intakes and of requirements. This can be considered in the framework of the relationship portrayed in Figure 1. Data on the observed usual intakes of food by the population may be translated to nutrient intake with the use of existing food composition data. A data bank, an appropriate coding system, and a computer program are required and could possibly be based upon one or more of the several systems now existing in the United States. However, for some nutrients, the nature of the food ingested and the total diet affect bioavailability. Reasonable information about the relationship between nature of the diet and relative bioavailability is available for a number of these nutrients.

Information about the individual's actual requirement is needed to determine the adequacy of intake relative to requirement. Clearly, such information is not available. With respect to the individual, the best estimate that can be made is the relative probability that the intake does or does not meet the individual's actual requirement. At a population level, using the bivariate distribution approach, an estimate can be made of the number of individuals (but not which individuals) with intakes below their actual requirements. The required data base for such estimates includes both the mean requirement for that category of individual and the variability of requirements among similar individuals. The *Recommended Dietary Allowances* (Food and Nutrition Board, 1980) is not an appropriate reference criteria* for these determinations, but, with current information, reasonable assumptions can be made about the distribution pattern for the requirements of a number of nutrients. Simplified analyses based on dietary scores or the use of indicator nutrients warrant further investigation to enhance the usefulness of the data for various purposes.

The preceding discussion has been related to the prediction of the prevalence of intakes below actual requirements of healthy individuals. The present information base relating "requirement" and level of nutritional status is fragmentary. It is germane to recognize that neither the meaning of "requirement," definition of the level of nutritional health to which the requirement applies, nor consideration of the degree of inadequacy of intake have been addressed in this discussion.

Information about the levels of intake required to maintain different levels of nutritional status is necessary if intakes are to be linked with observed severity or frequency of inadequate nutritional status. Lörstad (1974) has

*By definition, the "recommended dietary allowances" (RDA) as published by the Food and Nutrition Board are intended to be sufficiently high to cover the known nutritional needs of practically all healthy people. Therefore, RDA (except for energy) are estimated to exceed the requirements of most individuals. Intakes below the RDA are not necessarily inadequate, but the risk of inadequacy increases to the extent that intake is less than the level recommended as safe.

pointed out that with such information the same format of bivariate distribution analysis, with different requirement figures, could offer a series of predictions of the prevalence of different levels of nutritional status.

It would seem that, for many nutrients, there is now sufficient information to apply the bivariate system approach to the interpretation of dietary data. The information currently available may be imprecise and could certainly be improved with additional research. Nevertheless, for many nutrients, the quality of data available seems adequate to justify the assumptions about bioavailability, average requirements, distribution of requirements, and even requirements for different levels of nutritional status that are necessary for the statistical approach to analysis. Unfortunately, for some other nutrients there are major gaps in the information base that place analogous limitations on the above and other approaches to dietary data interpretation (Beaton *et al.*, 1979).

It is emphasized again that this approach does not make provision for effects of recurrent infection, of unusual environmental stress, of genetic abnormalities, of adaptabilities of host to excesses or deficiencies, or even of nutrient imbalances other than as they are built into estimates of bioavailability or requirement. This is a limitation of the model but one that should not preclude its use in the United States in a nutrition monitoring system.

Dietary data may also be used in the assessment of the probable risk associated with excessive, rather than inadequate, intakes of natural or added constituents of foods. The approach and data requirements are analogous. In this case, what will be needed are data pertaining to the average level of intake at which manifestations of harm are suspected (analogous to average requirements of a nutrient) and the possible variability of this sensitivity among individuals. As before, the probable prevalence of various grades/severities of toxicity (analogous to various levels of nutritional status) can be estimated if information is available on the relationship between level of intake and severity of the detrimental effect.

The bivariate analysis of dietary data, then, permits an examination of the population risks associated with both low and high intakes. It also permits an examination of the probable effects of a change in food consumption, such as a proposed food fortification policy or a proposed limit for a food additive, on intake and population risk. Implementation of this approach to analysis poses certain study design requirements and necessitates the compilation of certain data bases. These are discussed in some detail in later sections of the report.

As previously mentioned, predicting health status of individuals from dietary data alone is not possible. The role of certain foods or food components in the etiology of such chronic diseases as diabetes, coronary heart disease, atherosclerosis, hypertension, and cancer is not well documented (Ahrens and Conner, 1979). In addition, there appears to be a wide variation in the susceptibility of individuals within a population to these diseases. Knowledge concerning the relationship of food consumption patterns to susceptibility to chronic disease can better be determined from a careful examination of the food consumption patterns of population groups with known unusual incidences of these chronic diseases. Care must be taken to control adequately for environmental and genetic factors.

A number of the health-data bases in existence could be used in conjunction with food intake data to develop an appropriate monitoring system. Data from current health-data bases would need to be identified, summarized, and evaluated in those population subgroups used for food intake data analysis. Details are discussed in a later section of the report.

The Proposed System

It is proposed that an ongoing system be developed and implemented by the federal agencies with major interests in food consumption and health. This system should encompass these components or subsystems:

- A continuous collection, processing, and review of food intake data from a stratified probability sample of the U.S. population. This is the core of the food consumption data.
- The collection of health status indicator data from currently available sources and their collation for population strata analogous to those from which the dietary information is derived.
- The ongoing examination of available aggregate data from commercial and governmental sources on market food disappearance from regional and economic strata comparable to the above.

Collation, analysis, and reporting of information from these three subsystems should be the responsibility of a lead agency in the federal government. This agency must have adequate personnel and fiscal capability to undertake special purpose analyses of the data bases generated by the above subsystems. There should be provision also for government and non-government investigators, after appropriate review of requests, to have access to the data base for meritorious projects deemed to be in the public interest. The lead agency must also have the human and fiscal sources necessary to initiate or promote field studies or other specific investigative projects in response to food-health problems or potential problems revealed by the ongoing monitoring of the data system.

The system as outlined above, and the data bases so generated, will be capable of:

- monitoring the nutritional adequacy of the food practices and food supply of the general population;
- monitoring general health trends and their potential relationship to food usage;
- identifying sectors of the population in which particular food intake-related risks may be high and about which particular concerns should exist or in which special in-depth studies should be undertaken;
- providing a data base for testing probable effects of fortification programs, food additive regulations, nutritional standards or guidelines for food products, and similar federal needs;
- monitoring potential risk associated with selected food components or contaminants; and
- providing a sound data base for studies for the examination of relationships between food intake and chronic disease in segments of the U.S. population.

FOOD INTAKE OF INDIVIDUALS—SUBSYSTEM I

It is recommended that this subsystem be established as an ongoing operation, with rapid processing of data and with capability to collate and analyze data on a "moving average" basis.

The establishment of data collection, processing, and analysis as an ongoing operation will permit the responsible lead agency to develop and maintain a highly qualified unit operating on a continuous basis. The necessary experience in the various aspects of these operations can be highly developed and the unit fully employed on an ongoing basis. This will improve operational efficiency and eliminate administrative problems inherent in a system that is only periodically involved in such studies.

For purposes of sampling design, it is suggested that the time frame for collection of a statistically adequate sample of the stratified U.S. population be 5 years. It is recommended that the design provide for the collection and processing of these data at the rate of 20 percent of the full sample per year. It is recommended that analysis and interpretation be updated each year on the basis of data accumulated for the preceding 5 years (a moving 5-year average). The annual analysis also will provide trend information for the 12-month period as an "early warning" of developing problems. This system of sample collection is portrayed graphically in Figure 2.

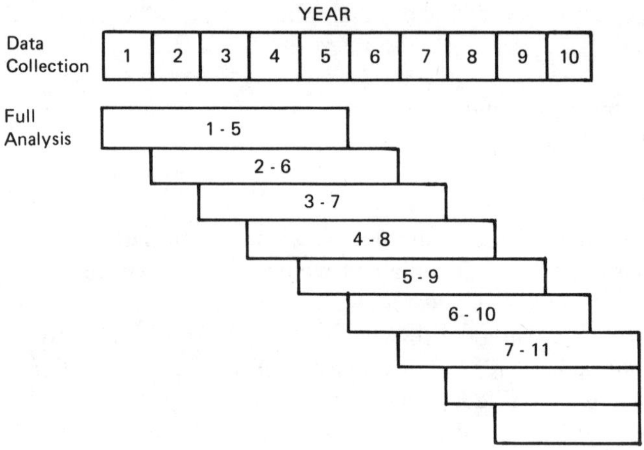

FIGURE 2 Time frame for sample collection.

Measurement of Food Intake

The data collection system should provide for replicated 1-day observations of the same individuals in sufficient number and stratification to provide an estimate of the distribution of usual intakes among the selected strata of the population. The recommended data collection technique is a 24-hour recall by trained interviewers using standardized instruments and food models to help respondents estimate quantity of food consumed and probe for precise information. This recall may be supplemented with a 3-day food record and a food frequency questionnaire to provide additional data concerning frequency of food use. The data collection and processing system must provide for internal quality control and should provide external validity checks as appropriate procedures are developed.

Four replicated 24-hour recall observations on the same individual within the 1-year sampling period may be necessary to provide a measure of the usual food intake of that individual (and of the variation currently experienced) adequate for use in determining the usual food intake pattern of the population group. Research should be initiated to determine the measurement frequency required for stipulated levels of reliability of the estimate of usual food intakes of individuals in a population and for estimation of the extremes of food consumption patterns. The precision required will vary with each study.

Sampling

The stratification of sampling should be designed to permit statistically reliable estimates of risks (low or high intake in comparison to actual needs

TABLE 1 Stratification of Sampling

Age and Physiologic State	Population Density	Region	Socioeconomic Level	Race and Ethnicity
0–5 yr	Metropolitan	Northeast	High	White
6–10 yr	Urban	Northwest	Middle	Black
11–20 yr	Periurban	Southeast	Low	Spanish-American
Male	Rural	Southwest	Poverty	Other
Female				
Pregnant				
Lactating				
21–45 yr				
Male				
Female				
Pregnant				
Lactating				
46–65 yr				
Male				
Female				
66+ yr				
Male				
Female				

or tolerances), as well as group averages. The population may be stratified, for example, according to the characteristics listed in Table 1.

It is recognized that it may not be feasible to design all of these and other desired features into a sampling frame and stratification design. It is also recognized that it will not be feasible to provide adequate numbers of individuals for distribution analyses in all cells potentially generated by the above 26 traits ($14 \times 4 \times 4 \times 4 \times 4 = 3{,}548$) and that in data analyses it will be necessary to collapse cells. Therefore, it is recommended that an experienced design group be charged with the development of an optimal design, taking into account first the questions to be put to the data and second the cost and logistical considerations. An auxiliary consideration in the sampling and analysis design should be the feasibility of collating health status indicator data for analogous subpopulations since it is the intent of the overall system that data from different sources be linked at the level of the subpopulation group and not at the level of individuals.

Data Base Requirements

It will be necessary to charge specific individuals or organizations with the development of requisite data bases for the proposed analysis system from existing information. These data bases will include distribution of nutrient requirements, distribution of food component tolerances, and food composition data including both nutrients and nonnutrients. A cooperative effort by government, academia, and industry will be needed. It is to be expected that over time the current data bases will improve in quality. The food consumption data base must be maintained in a format that permits recalculation of the intakes and reassessment of risks as other data bases improve or other needs for the data arise.

Coding and Data Analysis

The descriptors of consumed food that are entered and retained in the data base files must be sufficiently precise to allow answers for questions that may be posed at a later time. The descriptors are necessary even though information about food composition may not yet be available for all foods that can be precisely identified. While it would be desirable to identify manufacturers in food descriptions, such reporting would greatly expand the detail of the food coding system and the size of the data base storage requirement and, as a result, might reduce the reliability of data by increasing the chance of error. It is recommended that, as the system is developed, a special advisory group be convened to address the questions of precision of food identification and coding in the collection and storage of current and future food consumption data. These decisions must be made with an awareness of priority questions that are and will be put to the data base.

It seems probable that certain questions will not be answerable from the data base. For example, it may be difficult to generate reliable estimates of the distribution of intakes of infrequently used foods or of intakes of particular brands of foods. In these cases, the agency may choose to undertake specific consumption or frequency studies either as additions to dietary interviews proposed or as separate studies. The agency, on the other hand, may turn to other agency or commercial sources of data when these sources meet the requirements.

HEALTH STATUS INDICATOR DATA—SUBSYSTEM II

The stated objective of this system is to yield information that may be valuable in maintaining or improving the state of health, including nutritional status, of the U.S. population. Therefore, it is necessary to relate food consumption patterns to nutritional and health status. However, knowledge of the relationships between food consumption, nutritional status, and general health status is limited, and many areas are controversial. Careful examination of the factors to be studied and the data to be collected is required to ensure relevance to the issues under examination and to permit appropriate interpretation.

Existing health data bases can be used in conjunction with food intake data. While it is not necessary to collect both types of information from the same individuals, the collation, transfer, and summarization of health data according to population characteristics that can be duplicated in food consumption studies will be necessary.

The coordinated studies will focus initially on identified or postulated food-related health problems and will expand as relationships become clear. The health indicator data base should include information relevant to these acknowledged and possible relationships; however, there are practical limitations on the extent to which health conditions can or should be identified and retained in the data base of this subsystem.

Nutritional status is one component of health. From the proposed system, the usual food intake of individuals will be known, and this information can be used to estimate the risk of nutritional inadequacy (or excess) but not to identify the nutritional state or health of specific individuals. While prediction of the nutritional status of a population group can be assisted by limited use of anthropometric and biochemical measures, it is not recommended that this proposed monitoring system include these costly measurements for the total population sample. Rather, the collection of anthropometric data (such as height for weight, height for age, or height and weight for age) and biochemical measures (such as hemoglobin or hematocrit) should be limited to a population subsample. A detailed dietary and/or health history of individuals contacted for dietary recall information may, on occasion, be desirable. More detailed or extensive evaluations may be indicated if pilot studies identify prevalent problems in population segments.

In order to increase the potential for identifying relationships between food consumption and health status, it is recommended that available statistics be examined to identify population segments whose health indicators appear to be abnormal relative to the population average and to averages of other subgroups. Special studies of food consumption should be carried out in these population segments and/or an appropriate sampling of this population subgroup should be included in a regular monitoring program that combines information on diet and health.

Reliable statistics are available from many sources, but the data are not collated in the manner necessary to identify potential groups for study. It is recommended that a task force consider the existing sources of health information and the optimal approach to the identification and transfer of these data for use in the proposed system. The relationship of the health data to income status of population groups should also be evaluated to determine if, at least for some indicators, sampling based on economic stratification may yield the desired information. Identification of population segments to be studied should be made with a recognition of, first, the priority questions likely to be put to the composite data base, and second, the logistics and cost.

AGGREGATE FOOD DATA—SUBSYSTEM III

A number of sources of aggregate data on food disappearance and food purchase now exist within the government and the private sector. Some data are available at a national level only. Others provide data grouped according to regional or consumer characteristics. Sources in the private sector commonly provide information about specific commodities and specific brands and are designed to be rapidly responsive to market trends.

Comparison of aggregate food disappearance or food purchase data with the composite of food intake data over the time period should provide a basis for predicting relationships between the data bases. With this information, the aggregate data bases may prove to be very useful as an early warning component of the proposed system by detecting changes in foods reaching the consumer. They may be of additional use for special purpose studies, such as tracking specific commodities used in commercial products. It is recommended that uses of aggregate data bases to supplement information needed for a total overall monitoring system be identified.

IMPLEMENTATION OF THE TOTAL SYSTEM

Many parts of the proposed system, i.e., data bases and collection systems, already exist within various agencies of government. However, the parts have not been coordinated or applied as effectively as might be possible.

It is recommended that interagency discussions be undertaken with the objective of developing a coordinated system of the type described herein. Primary implementation responsibility should be assigned to one lead agency or to an interagency institution. This responsibility should relate not only to the coordination and analysis of data, but also to control of the quality of sampling, data collection, and data processing. The final conclusions can be no stronger than the weakest link between the unit that supplies information and the final processing of data to be examined.

Some Study Design Characteristics

DIETARY METHODOLOGY

Selection among available methods for assessing food and/or nutrient intake of households or individuals depends on available resources (funds, time, and personnel), the objectives of the study, and the target population (Marr, 1971). The effectiveness of any survey method in answering questions about food or nutrient intake of a population is contingent upon a statistically adequate sampling frame to assure that appropriate respondents are used and that oversampling of targeted groups to meet specific needs is permitted.

In general, information on food intake is obtained by (1) inference, (2) observation, and (3) verbal or written reports. Each has some inherent strengths and limitations, so a combination of methods may be needed.

Inferred data are derived primarily from aggregate data provided by commodity reports, commercial surveys of movement of food products in and out of warehouses or markets, and national food balance reports. These data provide information on trends in food consumption for a population group. They do not provide information on average intakes or ranges of intakes of individual consumers. Aggregate data can serve as a surrogate for individual data if the above limitations are understood. However, aggregate data are most useful in validating observations generalized to the total population from individual data.

Direct personal observation is generally so costly of money, time, and personnel that it is precluded in large-scale surveys and is used primarily to validate reported data. The observations may be either obtrusive (such as participant observation, which may in short-term studies result in modified behavior) or unobtrusive (such as monitoring store purchases and correlating them with specific individuals, which may constitute an invasion of privacy). Both modified behavior and invasion of privacy are serious obstacles to the use of methods involving observation of food intake.

As a result of the limitations of inferred and observed data, reporting is generally regarded as the most feasible and cost-effective way of learning about food intake of individuals and groups. Reported data are obtained by oral interview or are recorded by the subject. Oral interviews involve retrospective accounts with the interviewer available in person or by telephone. Food frequency information, a dietary history, and/or a 24-hour recall of food intake may be recorded by or for the subject in a written, telephoned, or tape-recorded format. Food intake records may be maintained in this manner for from one to usually no more than 7 days.

Usefulness of a reporting method depends on validity and reliability of the information reported, on the cost and speed of data collection and analysis, and on the appropriateness for both long- and short-range goals of the survey. Conclusions are only as good as the quality of the core information on which they are based, so an ongoing effort to assess the validity of the reported data is essential. Although there is considerable information on the reliability of various techniques for obtaining written and oral reports, there is very little information on validity of the data obtained. Limited studies done on small subsamples of the population indicate a tendency to underreport at upper levels of intake and to overreport at lower levels. This phenomenon, known as the "flat slope syndrome," casts doubt on the interpretation of data as regards extremes of intake. The extent to which actual and reported intakes vary appears to differ with the nutrient studied; therefore, the "flat slope syndrome" may need to be evaluated across the range of nutrients (Gersovitz *et al.*, 1978).

There is an urgent need for methodological studies for assessment of the validity of currently used dietary survey techniques in a range of circumstances and for identification and validation of alternative and innovative methods for obtaining food intake information (Garn *et al.*, 1978). While this report suggests four replications, questions remain regarding the minimum number of days or other units of time for which reported observations must be made in order to assess usual dietary intake and produce an accepted representation of actual intake. It has been reported in at least one study that validity of record keeping by adults decreases after 4 consecutive days (Gersovitz *et al.*, 1978). There does not seem to be a similar problem when records are kept for several days intermittently (Beaton *et al.*, 1979). Records of a single day's intake of individuals representing weekdays and weekend days over a long enough interval to detect cyclic changes have been found to give an acceptable estimate of usual food consumption

(Houser and Bebb, 1981). Probing to clarify records and enhance the accuracy of recall has resulted in substantial increases in the completeness of records (Campbell and Dodds, 1967). Analyses of food intake records using James–Stein indicators show that nutrient intakes regress toward the mean and that averages of 5 (and possibly fewer) days may give values that more closely approximate usual intakes than do individual day intakes (Samonds *et al.*, 1978). Other methodological questions for which there are only limited answers and which require further research are how to ensure immediate reporting, how to standardize estimates of serving sizes and descriptions of food items, the extent to which the homemaker can report for other family members, and the extent and nature of interviewer differences.

Written records are useful with literate, motivated subjects but not with those who are illiterate or poorly motivated or those with impaired vision or lack of neuromuscular coordination. Oral records are useful with these groups, but they often necessitate either a costly personal interview or the use of a recording device that may be technically baffling or too impersonal to encourage continued participation. Interviews that provide an opportunity for probing and permit clarification of food identification have been found to increase reported intakes by as much as 25 percent and to prolong participation, but they may encourage subjects to strive to respond in a perceived approved fashion.

A limited study of the validity of food records telephoned each day to a nutritionist or a telephone answering service showed them to be as valid as a 24-hour recall or a 7-day food record (Raker, 1979). Reports given to the nutritionist who could probe for some specific information were judged to be more valid than those from a recording device. The phone survey technique has the advantages of assuring that records are kept each day and of being equally applicable for literate and nonliterate subjects. However, telephone recordings have limitations similar to those of written records and limit the population surveyed to respondents who have telephones.

Currently available methods for determining food intake and the inherent advantages and disadvantages of each are shown in Table 2. Dietary methodologies must be refined to identify feasible methods of minimizing their present limitations and disadvantages.

ESTIMATION OF USUAL INTAKES

The preceding discussion has defined many of the limitations of current methods for measuring food consumption patterns of individuals and population groups. Most methods in current use collect data relating to finite periods of time, i.e., 1, 2, 3, or 7 days. For the proposed system it will be necessary to collect data that describe the distribution of usual food intakes

TABLE 2 Dietary Survey Methodology

General Methods	Types of Information	Advantages	Disadvantages
1. *Inference*	Food balance Food disappearance Commodity reports	Tracks trends in food consumption Inexpensive	No information on individual or subgroup data Monitors only food in formal distribution system and commodity foods
2. *Observations*			
(A) Unobtrusive	TV monitoring	Minimal behavior modification	Invasion of privacy
	Use of grocery sale slips	May identify related social variables	Represents observed period only Grocery sale slips offer no way to assess distribution within household nor do they measure food from other sources
(B) Obtrusive	Participant observer	Identification of related factors	Behavior is modified Costly Represents one point in time
3. *Reported*			
(A) Oral interview—in person or by telephone (Retrospective information)	Food frequency Dietary history	Can be quantified Identifies limits of use Describes long-term and usual practices Applicable to group data	Requires long list and many judgments Difficult to quantify Difficult to integrate with other data

		Can probe for missing data	Costly
	24-hour recall	Can be quantified No opportunity to modify behavior Relatively short recall period Can probe for missing data	Requires good memory Desire to please interviewer alters recall Represents intake at one period—not usual intake
(B) Recorded by subject as written record, tape recorder, or by telephone	Food intake records 1 day 3 days 7 days to 28 days	Inexpensive Possible to build in mechanisms to assure immediate responses	Depends on ability to keep record Cooperation and validity decrease with time Record keeping can be delayed with longer time periods decreasing activity Less accurate information on food and amount
	Menu census 14 days	Detailed information on food taken into household and how it is used	Recorder may be unable to answer for all family members No data on food from other sources
(C) Weighed records	Actual weight of food consumed	High degree of accuracy	Respondents change behavior due to effect of observation

of the population group over an extended period of time. Statistically, this measure may be described as an estimate of the inter individual (between individual) variation. The relationship between observed variance and inter- and intraindividual variances is described by the following equation:

$$o^2 = o_b^2 + o_w^2/n,$$

where o^2 = observed variance, o_b^2 = interindividual (between individual) variance, o_w^2 = intraindividual (within individual) variance, and n = number of repeated observations for each individual. The last term (o_w^2/n) may be described as day-by-day variation in the intake of individuals. The magnitude of this component of variance may be estimated if the study design includes repeated measurements of 1-day intake for all, or an approximate representative sample of the individuals. Preferably these replications of 1-day data should be independent of one another (e.g., 1-day observations separated in time), but, with appropriate statistical treatment, related observations (e.g., the individual days of a 3-day record) may be used in estimating the intraindividual variance. The design should include appropriate sampling to measure the influence of seasons, holidays, and weekends on the patterns of food intake.

With knowledge of total or observed variance and of intraindividual variance, an estimate of interindividual variance (the measure of variation in *usual* intake) can be derived from the above equation. Repeated observations on the same individuals is the preferred method for measuring usual pattern of intake and its variation.

The reliability of the estimate of o_w^2 is a function of the total number of repeated 1-day observations. From the statistical point of view, collecting data from 100 people twice or 50 people three times (each pattern has 100 repeated days) leads to similar confidence limits in the estimate of intraindividual variance as long as the subjects observed are representative of the population. The decision on the desirable number of replications per subject should involve consideration of the logistics of repetitive examinations separated in time (i.e., as independent observations). The decision on the total number of additional measurements (total replications) must be based upon a consideration of needed confidence.

Since interindividual variance is calculated from intraindividual variation and observed total variance, it follows that if the total sample is large and hence the total variance has been reliably measured, the confidence of the estimate of interindividual variation is inversely related to the ratio of intra/interindividual variation. That is, as the magnitude of intraindividual variation increases in relationship to interindividual variation, the reliability of the estimate of intraindividual variation, and hence the number of replicate 1-day intake estimates required for the population must increase if a reliable estimate of interindividual variation is to be obtained. The statistical problem of confidence limits is considered in survey design.

Beaton and co-workers (1979) have provided estimates of the partitioning of variance for several nutrient sectors. It is apparent that this varies with the nutrient and with the food item under study. Thus, design requirements are a function of questions to be asked of the data.

It is extremely important that all sources of consumed food, including food supplements, alcoholic and nonalcoholic beverages, water, and medications, be incorporated into the data. The several methods for collecting individual food consumption data should be evaluated. In practice, no one method is likely to be perfect; therefore, it is necessary to select and adapt the best method to meet the needs of the particular study to be undertaken. Combinations of 24-hour recall with two or more 3-day diet records, food frequency questionnaires, telephone interviews, and/or extended diary records could be considered.

It should be remembered, however, that for the proposed monitoring system, repeated observations that permit measurement of the usual food intake and the extremes or variation by and between individuals are essential components. Internal quality control checks must be an integral part of this or any system. Validity checks are extremely important and a concerted effort should be made to develop and implement procedures to determine the validity of various methods of assessing dietary intake, including combinations of methods. Research is required to develop satisfactory systems for determining the validity of measurements obtained.

ASSESSMENT OF NUTRITIONAL STATUS

The conventional method of determining nutritional status of individuals and population groups relies primarily on biochemical assessment. The proposed food consumption monitoring system can provide only a probability estimate of nutritional status of a population group (by comparison of the usual nutrient intake with appropriate nutrient requirement figures). It is not possible from consumption data alone to identify the specific individuals in the population who are in a particular nutritional state.

Both prevalence and severity of nutritional inadequacy and excess are of concern in population assessment. In biochemical assessment, different levels of nutrients (in cells, tissues, and fluids) are associated with different probabilities of impaired function. Frequently, cutoff points are selected for categorization of deficiency or excess. As the cutoff point for adequacy is raised or lowered, the prevalence of deficiency appears to increase or decrease. However, it is the interpretation that has changed, not the prevalence or severity of functional impairment.

It is possible to establish a series of cutoff points related to the deficiency (or excess) of a nutrient, and it is possible to develop a series of prediction curves expressing the expected prevalence of varying degrees of deficiency (or excess) in the population. This can be done with biochemical data and with combination dietary and nutrient requirement data. Using the proposed system of estimating usual nutrient intake from usual food intake and relating this to usual nutrient requirement, information obtained from dietary data ought to be similar in accuracy to information obtained from biochemical data. When the estimates of nutritional adequacy indicate the probability that a particular population segment has a significant prevalence of inadequacy (or excess) for one or more nutrients, it may be desirable to study that population group in greater detail. Such studies must include biochemical assessment if the intent is to identify specific individuals who are in poor nutritional state.

RELATIONSHIP OF FOOD CONSUMPTION PATTERNS TO HEALTH STATUS INDICATORS

The possible relationship between food consumption patterns and health status provides the rationale for FDA interest in monitoring food consumption. Yet the relationships are complex and not easily documented. This section will attempt to provide some perspective on the types of indices and methods used in the proposed system, which will give a picture of food-related differences in health status in the population.

Three types of relationships between food consumption and health status are of concern. Firstly, health status is affected by food consumption through the intervening variable, nutritional state. For these types of health outcomes, dietary data have predictive value in population terms even though they are not direct measures of nutritional status. Selection of specific measures of nutritional status depends on the level of sensitivity required, e.g., degree of iron saturation.

A second type of relationship is one in which consumption of specific foods, substances, or combinations of these is linked to health status but not through the intervening variable, nutritional status. Most toxicological problems that are due to chance contamination of a specific production lot of a food are of this type. For this kind of linkage to be monitored effectively, it is essential that the food consumption data base be adaptable to very fine disaggregation by specific commodity product type, brand, or other factors. For some of these relationships, special *ad hoc* studies will have to be undertaken as the information required is likely to be highly specific to certain foods or population segments.

Food consumption patterns and/or nutritional status can also be contributing or facilitating factors but not the sole etiologic factor in the pathogenesis of diseases such as coronary heart disease, hypertension, or other chronic degenerative diseases. This third kind of relationship is characteristic of several of the leading causes of morbidity and mortality in the United States. Generally, the contributory role of diet is not well quantified. However, since diet may be the only factor that can be easily manipulated, it is important to know if differences in food consumption are associated with differing incidences of these diseases. In making this determination, it is important to control the other variables (such as heredity, occupation, etc.) known to affect the disease.

Irrespective of which of the three types of relationship is postulated, the disease or condition of concern must meet certain basic criteria (Institute of Medicine, 1973), which include the following:

1. have significant functional impact on those affected;
2. be relatively well defined and easy to diagnose in clinical and nonclinical settings;
3. have a prevalence rate that is high enough to permit the collection of adequate data from a limited population sample;
4. have a natural history that varies with utilization or consumption of food and/or nutrients; and
5. have potential for documentation of influences of nondietary variables.

Identification of a clear relationship between food consumption and health status indicators will suggest means of dietary intervention for prevention, and often treatment.

A systematic approach for relating a health status problem to food consumption data is essential. A logical progression of steps for such linkage is given below, recognizing that modification will be appropriate for specific conditions. There are six steps, which may be concurrent:

1. conducting retrospective studies to establish increased relative risk of disease (or decrement in a health status indicator) associated with differences in food consumption;
2. monitoring populations which have a particularly high or low prevalence or incidence of the disease indicator;
3. verifying the continued association in identified populations;
4. identifying populations with food consumption patterns indicating they may be at risk and initiating prospective studies in these populations in order to confirm the relationship and determine proportion of risk attributable to food consumption;

5. monitoring food consumption patterns of populations to detect those populations at risk; and
6. developing and implementing intervention strategies.

For some conditions, in particular acute and chronic toxicities, steps 2 to 5 may not be needed before intervention is undertaken. In cases where the association between health status and food consumption is firmly established, steps 1 to 4 may not be necessary. However, the general model provides a framework for an orderly approach to development of cost-effective intervention strategies.

Retrospective studies to establish an association of health status with food consumption are dependent on identifying probable associations through laboratory, clinical, or epidemiological studies. Appropriate study design must consider variables other than food consumption that may be related to the etiology or expression of the health state. Dietary methodologies described earlier will be used to determine current food consumption and to test its relationship to acute toxicities, perinatal events, infant morbidity or mortality, and the like. Different methodology is required to determine long-term food consumption patterns and their effect upon chronic toxicities, chronic disease, growth, etc. A projected need to use data generated by the proposed consumption monitoring system for this determination would have significant design and sampling implications.

An important aspect of the proposed system for relating food consumption to health status involves the use of existing health data on identified population segments to determine unusual health patterns. The usual pattern of food intake of these populations can then be determined in a special study or by oversampling the identified segment in the ongoing survey.

Health and food intake data are preferably obtained from the same individuals. If this is not possible, data should be collected on individuals of the same sample cell characteristics to provide as close a relationship as possible between usual food intake information and health status. When indications of a relationship between patterns of usual food intake and health status in a population group are observed, confirmation may be necessary through the use of special studies to obtain significant measures of nutritional and health status. Biochemical and anthropometric data as well as extensive dietary and medical histories of the individuals in the population under study may be required.

Data Base Requirements

The proposed monitoring and evaluation system requires the use of sources of data on food composition, nutrient requirements, aggregate food disappearance, and health. There is considerable variation in the adequacy of these data sources. The information may be incomplete, inaccurate, and out of date. It is necessary, however, to deal with the data that are available as the cost of collecting new data specifically for use in the proposed system would be prohibitive. There must be a continuing effort to upgrade these basic data sources in terms of quantity and quality of information and ease of access for use. This chapter discusses the sources required and many of the limitations that exist in the information they currently provide.

FOOD COMPOSITION DATA

The U.S. Department of Agriculture maintains the most extensive bank of data on food composition. The quantity and quality of the data are variable and in the case of many of the less studied nutrients are not adequate for an accurate calculation of nutrient intake.

Data for the nutrients for which need has long been established are relatively complete for food commodities. Data are much less complete for commercially prepared items, although much more information is becoming available as a result of nutrition labeling of many food products. For a number of the nutrients for which dietary requirements have more recently been identified, analytical data are fragmentary. For some nutrients, including several of the trace elements, content in food varies extensively with geographic region and growing conditions. Therefore, meaningful analytical descriptions may be difficult. However, when interest is in usual intake and hence usual composition, sample-to-sample variation in composition or small differences attributable to various processing or preparation practices may not be of concern.

For some studies, data on the composition of particular brands; changes caused by processing, packaging, and storage; and variations in composition due to changes in selection of ingredients (such as type of fat) may be required. In other studies, information on the composition of the water added to or used in preparation of the food items may be desirable. This type of information is very limited.

Conventional tables of food composition do not provide information about amounts of nonnutritive food additives or food contaminants present. If concern exists as to potential toxicity of any nonnutritive components or if dietary data are to be applied for prediction of risk of excessive intake, an increased data base describing the levels or potential levels in food is needed. Information on additive content in foods is currently available from GRAS (additives Generally Regarded As Safe) survey data prepared by the Committee on GRAS List Survey, Phase III, Food and Nutrition Board, the Food and Drug Administration, and other sources.

As the needs of each study are different, decisions on the desirable detail of description of foods must be made at the time of data collection. It is, however, necessary to keep in mind potential future uses for the data.

The incomplete nature of available data banks currently limits the attainment of accurate and useful nutrient intake data. Current data bases must be expanded to include some information on formulated, processed, and ethnic foods as well as mass-produced fast food items and products prepared for institutional use. More data on a wider number of nutrients for many foods should be provided.

The ideal data base would (1) be current, reliable, and valid; (2) be responsive to changes in the food supply; (3) contain information on all the nutrients of interest; (4) have complete data (unavailable data should be extrapolated until analytical values are obtained); (5) be expandable as new data become available; (6) reflect differences associated with brands; and (7) be in a physical form that facilitates coding and analysis.

Coding System

Concurrent with the further development of data banks for nutrient analysis must be the development of a coding system that will allow maximum flexibility in analyzing data and identifying and tracking trends in food consumption patterns. Coding by the various food consumption data banks must be standardized so information from several sources can be efficiently and easily combined. The coding system must be designed to mesh with health data systems. Simplified analyses based on dietary scores or the use of indicator nutrients warrant further investigation to enhance the usefulness of the data for various purposes.

Nutrient Requirement Estimates

It is customary in evaluating data on dietary intake to compare calculated nutrient intakes to the Food and Nutrition Board's Recommended Dietary Allowances (RDA). This practice leads to misinterpretation of nutrient intake data. Intake data may be interpreted more accurately by a bivariate distribution approach that requires a description of the distribution of nutrient requirements (median plus variance). For many nutrients, these data are available. For other nutrients, appropriate informed judgment can be made about the distribution of requirements and, thus, the extent of variance. For a few nutrients, there are insufficient data to permit even an informed judgment, and interpretation of observed intake is not possible.

It will be necessary to compile existing data and prepare descriptions of the distributions of nutrient requirements. Therefore, data on average requirements and their variances should be collected and published. At the same time it will be necessary to aggregate data on nutrient requirements for different levels of nutritional status if an assessment of both prevalence and severity of nutritional risk is to be made. Such data are available for many nutrients. For example, the average requirement of thiamin to prevent neurological manifestations of deficiency is estimated to be about 0.20–0.22 mg/1,000 kcal (FAO/WHO, 1967). The average requirement for physiologic saturation of tissue needs, judged by the pattern of urinary excretion, is about 0.33 mg/1,000 kcal with a coefficient of variation of requirement of 10 percent of the mean (FAO/WHO, 1967). Data are now available relating thiamin intake to erythrocyte transketolase activity. These types of information provide estimates of requirements for different levels of nutritional status and can be used in the bivariate distribution analysis. Thus, in attempting to relate dietary status to health status, it is necessary to express requirement in terms of purpose: e.g., prevention of clinical deficiency, maintenance of a level of enzyme activity, etc. To what extent all of these criteria relate to health status remains to be determined.

AGGREGATE DATA

A number of "food use" government and commercial data systems currently collect data on a continuing or periodic basis. These data series can be classified by the degree of aggregation of the data that they present and, therefore, by the applications to which they can be put. Avenues for their effective use in conjunction with individual data should be identified.

Production and shipment data are usually collected from the producers or the distributors of the raw commodities of the processed foods. The primary source of agricultural output data is the U.S. Department of Agriculture. Other sources include the Department of Commerce, the Bureau of Census, various growers or manufacturer associations, the state agricultural departments, and the alcoholic beverage production and tax control commissions of the states and the federal government. Most of these data are published in standardized time series.

Warehouse withdrawal data are collected from the data processing records of large warehouses of supermarket chains, or food and grocery product brokers. The data are aggregated and reported for a large number of markets or cities. Information is presented on individual brands, by type of product, by size of package, and for canned, packaged, refrigerated, and frozen foods. Most fresh fruits and vegetables, fresh meat, and similar items that do not move through the chain warehouses or the computerized inventory management systems of the stores are not included. The data are usually reported in raw unprojected form, covering sales in each market for the cooperating chains. The system in many areas accounts for 50 to 75 percent of all foods sold. The information is usually sold to food manufacturers and advertisers on a product-class basis for confidential use and not for resale or publication. Standard reports are usually issued, but customized processing is possible.

Audits of in-store movement of food items are made by a number of commercial services. These services collect their information from a selected sample of supermarkets throughout the United States. A physical audit of the quantities of various products on the shelf and delivered into each store is made bimonthly. This information is then projected from the sample to total market levels and aggregated into regional subtotals and a U.S. total. Per-capita availability can be determined from these audits and warehouse withdrawal data.

Aggregated consumer food purchase and usage data are collected by consumer purchase panels. These syndicated data services collect information via the mail from continuing nationwide samples of households and project these data to regional and U.S. totals. Diaries are collected from consumers weekly or monthly. Occasionally, custom samples are set up in selected cities for test marketing purposes, operated for a period of from ½ to 2 years, and then disbanded. Consumer records include mail-order, door-to-door, and specialty store purchases in addition to grocery store purchases. Reports are issued to subscribers on a monthly or quarterly basis. Reports include data on the total quantity of the product bought, the average price paid, the percent of households by which the product was bought, and the average quantity bought per buying household. Data on consumption by individuals within the household are not provided.

A "Menu Census Service" provides detailed information on food preparation and on all food consumed at and away from home from regional or nationwide samples. Data are collected by mail following maintenance of consecutive days of diaries of individual food intake. Data for each food product are summarized and reported quarterly and annually. Usage of each food product is cross-tabulated by the demographic characteristics of the household and the individual eaters. Persons living away from home or in institutions (i.e., schools, hospitals, armed forces) are not included in consumer purchase panels or menu census services.

Food consumption surveys of selected products or sources are conducted by various companies. The data are collected by mail from consumers on a continuing syndicated basis. Information on, for example, the consumption of all foods at restaurants, or the consumption of all beverages at home or away from home, is summarized into standard reports designed to satisfy selected information needs of a given industry, such as soft drink manufacturers or restaurant operators.

HEALTH STATUS DATA BASES

Indicators of health status are objective measures of the state of health of a population. Health status indicators with a nutritional status component fall into several categories comprising the continuum from "perfect" health to death from a variety of illnesses and disease. The first category, morbidity, includes specific diseases with an apparent nutritional component and ones where evaluation of nutritional status would provide an indication of potential risk of the disease. Among these diseases, but not limited to them, are noninsulin-dependent diabetes, atherosclerosis, hypertension, cirrhosis of the liver, gout, osteoporosis, obesity, coronary heart disease, dental disease, anemia, cerbrovascular disease, and, possibly, cancer. Of less importance, but still significant, would be others, including gastrointestinal disorders, respiratory disease, a variety of conditions subsumed within aging, nutrient inadequacy and toxicity, chance contaminations, and food-borne illnesses.

The next group of health status indicators may be drawn from mortality statistics. Of particular nutritional importance are infant mortality, perinatal mortality, and age-specific mortality rates indicative of longevity.

The third group are those indicators that are characteristics of the population and are nutrition related. They include the incidence of low birth weight, the age at menarche, the outcome of early adolescent pregnancies, birth defects, obesity, stunted growth, and behavioral or functional conditions (including those related to learning and to performance).

Nutritional status indicators are considered a category of health status indicators. They include the various types of measures by which nutritional status is determined: (1) biochemical (including blood and urine samples), (2) anthropometric, and (3) clinical (including behavioral measures). The data derived from such measurements are used in two ways: to identify individuals at risk who may then be recalled for follow-up examinations, and to identify groups that are at risk and design appropriate programs to alleviate the risk. Nutritional status determinations are complex, time-consuming, and expensive.

The methodology of relating food consumption to information on health, including nutrition status indicators, encompasses a range of data-gathering, coding, and analytical procedures. The general types of food consumption information desired for useful analyses can be divided into three groups:

1. Feeding behavior, which includes the pattern of meals within a family, the type of infant feeding, the frequency of eating, the proportion and location of meals eaten outside the home, snacking patterns, food preparation, and many others;
2. Food groupings, which can be as finely divided as the investigator thinks necessary;
3. Food components: saturated and unsaturated fats, cholesterol, sugars, other carbohydrates, fiber, animal and vegetable proteins, specific nutrients, additives and contaminants.

Some aspects of a system for relating food consumption to health status do exist, but the linkages can seldom be made due to inconsistencies in methods and in populations studied. Existing information is often not fully used, and studies are not often compatible with existing information sources or with other new studies.

Monitoring for the conditions in populations can be at several levels and may utilize already existing health or individual data or may require field survey methods. Table 3 indicates sources of information currently available on defined populations of suitable size to detect small area or regional differences. The sources of information are varied, at present are not integrated, may be redundant, and have varying degrees of validity. Development of these information sources into a complementary, if not single, information system should be undertaken.

Medical record linkage as a method to utilize the diverse sources of information should be developed. Such development will require that current concern about privacy and confidentiality of personal records be satisfactorily resolved in favor of the ability to carry out epidemiologic studies.

TABLE 3 Types and Sources of Health Status Data

Vital Statistics	*Health Screening Program*
Birth records	Voluntary agencies
National Center for Health Statistics	Public health agencies
Death records	*Disease Registries*
National Center for Health Statistics	Voluntary agencies
Linked birth and death records	Public health agencies
Public health agencies	*School Health Records*
Special studies	*Population Surveys*
Medical Records	National Health Survey
Hospital discharge data	Special studies
Commission on Professional and Hospital Activities	*Epidemic Intelligence*
Professional Standards Review Organization	Centers for Disease Control
Insurance data banks	Public health agencies
Tumor registry	
National data set	
Local registries	
Physician records	
Group practices	
National Disease and Therapeutic Index	
Insurance Claims	
Institutions	

Appropriate safeguards against invasion of privacy and breach of confidentiality must be built into the system in such a way that linkage is not proscribed.

At present there is a vast amount of information on mortality and morbidity in existing computer tapes. Most of the types of data shown in Table 3 are currently collected and stored in accessible form. There is a need for new ideas and methods to utilize these data sources in combination with food consumption data in defined populations. For example, fetal nutritional experience seems to offer an excellent prospect for studying chronic disease within a realistic time cycle. Surveillance of various indices of infant birth and mortality, linked to birth certificate data, and study of these data in a comprehensive way could shorten the long observation periods needed to collect mortality and morbidity perspectively in adult populations (Hawthorne, 1981).

For purposes of illustration, certain selected conditions considered at present to be strongly associated with food consumption are listed in Table 4. The types and sources of health data that could be utilized in population

TABLE 4 Health Status Indicator Data Associated with Food Consumption

Age Group	Condition	Vital Statistics	Medical Records	Screening Programs	Disease Registries	School Records	Surveys	Epidemic Intelligence
Infants	Perinatal mortality	x						
	Low birth weight	x						
	Fetal alcohol syndrome		x					
	Physical development						x	
Children	Growth		x				x	
	Mental development					x		
	Anemia			x			x	
	Hyperlipidemia		x	x			x	
	Caries		x	x		x	x	
Adults	Obesity		x	x			x	
	Hypertension	x	x	x	x		x	
	Diabetes	x	x	x	x		x	
	Neoplasia, specific	x	x	x	x			
	Acute toxicity		x					x
	Chronic toxicity	x	x				x	

studies are indicated in the table. While the sources vary in the degree of validity of the data contained in them, they form a rich pool of information for assessment of the health of populations.

The many health data files that exist in the United States should be cataloged and those that may provide data for relating health status to food consumption patterns identified. It is recommended that a special work group be established to evaluate current health statistical information and recommend a system whereby these data can be collated in a manner that will permit identifying population segments showing unusual health patterns. Once identified, the integration of this information with the proposed system for monitoring food consumption patterns should be developed. In this manner studies can be targeted to specifically identified groups either through special studies or as a part of the ongoing monitoring program.

If information on food consumption and nutritional status were obtained in a compatible format, this system could be used to explore associations between food consumption and health status, while taking into account the modifying effect of other factors.

There is a current need in the United States for specific information on food consumption and health status (obtained at the same time and from the same individuals) in order to identify specific associations. There is an additional need to obtain this type of information in a consistent manner, on the same individual as often as possible, and at repeated time intervals in order to detect trends and changes over time.

Conclusions and Recommendations

The Food and Drug Administration has need of reliable data concerning individual food consumption. These data are important for adequate assessment of the safety and wholesomeness of the U.S. food supply, for assessment of the effect of incidental contaminants and food additives, and for development of food fortification policies and nutritional quality criteria for food products. FDA must also be concerned with putative linkages between food consumption patterns and health. An ability to forecast the effect of changes in food consumption patterns on nutrient intake and on health and productivity would aid the agency in formulation of sound policies and programs with respect to food fortification, consumer education, nutrition and food intervention, and the like. In the final analysis, the need for food consumption data stems from concern for health promotion and prevention of adverse health response in the population.

Systems currently in use in the United States do not meet the needs of FDA. While the system proposed in this report is intended to meet the specific needs of FDA, it may well prove useful to other government agencies and institutions engaged in monitoring food consumption, nutritional status, and health.

The proposed system is based on continuous determination of the usual pattern of food intake of individuals and population groups. This information plus information on variation in food intakes and food composition data can be used to determine the usual pattern of nutrient intake and its variation. It is not possible from dietary data alone to assess nutritional status. However, it is possible, with current knowledge of human requirements, to assess the individual's risk of inadequate status based on intake of certain nutrients—and to predict for a normally distributed population the prevalence of individuals who have intakes below requirements. It is also possible to estimate the risk of excessive intake of nutrients and of natural or added food components, if there is knowledge of the association between level of intake and risk of toxicity.

The health and nutritional status of individuals cannot be predicted from dietary data alone. However, if dietary data can be linked to existing health data, health status indicators believed to be associated with food or nutrient intake can be identified. Data from appropriate studies of the food consumption patterns of individuals in a group could then be used to predict the prevalence of individuals with increased risk to health from a particular pattern of food or nutrient intake.

Economic considerations and other factors may influence decisions as to adoption of the proposed system. In addition, certain data bases are not currently adequate. However, the Committee believes the method proposed is sound and information gathered thereby would be significantly better than that derived from methods that are currently in use.

The Committee recommends that an ongoing system be developed and implemented by the federal agencies that have major interests in food consumption and health. The system should encompass the following components or subsystems:

- a continuous collection, processing, and review of food intake data from a stratified probability sample of consumption data;
- the collection of health data from currently available sources and their collation for population strata analogous to those from which dietary information is derived; and
- ongoing examination of available aggregate data from commercial and governmental sources on market food disappearance, from regional and economic strata comparable to the above.

Ideally, a lead federal agency should take responsibility for collating, analyzing, and reporting information from these three subsystems. This agency must have adequate personnel and fiscal resources to undertake special data analyses as needed.

Several areas require special consideration for implementation of an efficient and reliable system. The Committee recommends that research be initiated to determine the measurement frequency required for stipulated levels of reliability of the estimate of usual food intakes of individuals in a population and for estimation of the extremes of food consumption patterns. A group experienced in design should be charged with the development of an optimal sampling frame and stratification design to meet the needs of the system.

Several data bases require further development. It will be necessary to assign responsibility to specific individuals or organizations to develop the requisite data base from existing information. The Committee makes the following specific recommendations for the establishment of the proposed system:

1. This system be established as an ongoing operation, capable of rapid data processing and of collating and analyzing data on a continuing ("moving average") basis.
2. As the system is developed, a special advisory group be convened to address the question of precision of food identification and coding in the collection and storage of current and future food consumption data.
3. In order to increase the potential for identifying meaningful relationships between food consumption and health status, available statistics be examined to identify population segments whose health indicators appear to be abnormal relative to the population average and to the average of other subgroups.
4. A task force consider the existing sources of health status information and devise an effective approach to the identification and transfer of data to the proposed system.
5. The uses of aggregate data bases to supplement information needed for a total overall monitoring system be identified.
6. Interagency discussions be undertaken with the objective of developing a coordinated system.

References

Ahrens, E. H., and W. E. Conner, eds. 1979. Report of the task force on the evidence relating six dietary factors to the nation's health. Symposium sponsored by the American Society for Clinical Nutrition, Inc. Am. J. Clin. Nutr. (Suppl.) 32:2621–2748.

Beaton, G. H. and L. D. Swiss. 1974. Evaluation of the nutritional quality of food supplies: Prediction of "desirable" or "safe" protein: calorie ratios. Am. J. Clin. Nutr. 27:484–504.

Beaton, G. H., J. Milner, P. Corey, V. McGuire, M. Cousins, and J. A. Little. 1979. Sources of variance in 24-hour dietary recall data: Implications for nutrition study design and interpretation. Am. J. Clin. Nutr. 32:2546–2559.

Campbell, V. A., and M. L. Dodds. 1967. Collecting dietary information from groups of older people. J. Am. Diet. Assoc. 51:29–33.

Department of Health and Human Services. 1980. Promoting health/preventing disease: Objectives for the nation. U.S. Government Printing Office. Washington, D.C. 102 pp.

FAO/WHO. 1967. Report of the Joint FAO/WHO Expert Group. Requirement for vitamin A, thiamine, riboflavin, and niacin. WHO Tech. Rep. Ser. No. 362.

FAO/WHO. 1973. Report of the Joint FAO/WHO Ad Hoc Expert Committee. Energy and protein requirements. FAO Nutr. Meet. Rep. Ser. No. 522, WHO Tech. Rep. Ser. No. 522.

Food and Nutrition Board. 1980. Recommended Dietary Allowances, 9th ed. National Academy of Sciences/National Research Council, Washington, D.C. 185 pp.

Garn, S., F. A. Larkin, and P. E. Cole. 1978. The real problem with one-day records. Am. J. Clin. Nutr. 31:1114–1117.

General Accounting Office. 1978. Future of the national nutrition intelligence system. Study by the staff of the U.S. General Accounting Office. CED-79-5, November 7, 1978. 39 pp.

Gersovitz, M., J. P. Madden, and H. Smiciklas-Wright. 1978. Validity of 24-hour dietary recall and seven-day record for group comparisons. J. Am. Diet. Assoc. 73:48–55.

Hawthorne, V. M. 1981. In this volume.

Houser, H. B., and H. T. Bebb. 1981. In this volume.

Institute of Medicine. 1973. A strategy for evaluating health services. II. Contrasts in health status. National Academy of Sciences/National Research Council, Washington, D.C. 219 pp.

Lörstad, M. 1971. Recommended intake and its relation to nutrient deficiency. FAO Nutr. Newsl. 9(1): 18–31.

Lörstad, M. 1974. On estimating incidence of undernutrition. FAO Nutr. Newsl. 12(1):1–11.

Marr, J. W. 1971. Individual dietary surveys: Purposes and methods. World Rev. Nutr. Diet. 13:105.

Office of Science and Technology Policy, Executive Office of the President. 1977. New directions in federally supported human nutrition research. Nutrition Research Interagency Working Group, Washington, D.C. pp. 1–27.

Office of Technology Assessment, Congress of the United States. 1978. Nutrition research alternatives. U.S. Government Printing Office, Washington, D.C. 77 pp.

Raker, M. 1979. Validity of telephone food record. Unpublished master's thesis. The Pennsylvania State University.

Samonds, K. W., K. Donato, and D. M. Hegsted. 1978. The use of James-Stein estimators in the evaluation of nutrition survey data. Fed. Proc. 37:845. (Abstr.)

Swiss, L. D., and G. H. Beaton. 1974. A prediction of the effects of iron fortification. Am. J. Clin. Nutr. 27:373–379.

White House Conference on Food, Nutrition and Health. 1969. U.S. Government Printing Office, Washington, D.C. 341 pp.

APPENDIX

A Background Papers for Workshop on Methods for the Collection of Aggregate Data on Food Consumption

The Food System: An Overview

HAROLD F. BREIMYER

The extensive data that have been amassed and replenished regarding U.S. agriculture and the food system originated in large measure from the needs of operating programs. Their instigation with respect to, among others, food consumption data was more practical or programmatic than intellectual.

The emerging agricultural programs of the 1930's revealed a need for national statistics of many kinds that gave impetus to statistical collection programs that have long since been divorced from anything farmlike or rural. I joined the Agricultural Adjustment Administration in May 1936 and found economists there worrying about national income statistics and elasticity of demand for oranges and the effect of overseas trade, all with a sobriety never known to classroom academicians. I doubt George Jasny in the Department of Commerce has any idea how much the old operating agency of the Triple-A contributed to the national income data series over which he has exercised fatherly care for so long. Although the National Bureau of Economic Statistics properly gets the first credit for pioneering, I remember vividly how national income estimates of the department were spliced with the figures of the young Simon Kuznets in trying to arrive at some background statistical underpinning of demand estimates for farm products.

And so it was with data on food production and consumption. To be sure, from its beginning in 1862 the U.S. Department of Agriculture had compiled certain data on production of farm products. These had gradually been augmented with statistics arising from a variety of sources. Although certain marketing service activities had been carried on for a long time and market news reporting became an early fixture, many of the data can only be described as of happenstance origin. For example, early in our century, Upton

Sinclair set in motion popular support for meat inspection, as the public and especially export buyers did not like to know about workers falling into open-manhole lard-rendering vats. Once federal meat inspection activities were well under way, the managers of the agency had a natural desire to collect and report the figures on how much work they were doing. Therein commenced a series of data on production of federally inspected meat, which could readily be converted into carcass weight data on how much federally inspected meat was being consumed.

I remember well a meeting in the USDA when the meat inspection people decided they were being "had" as they performed a major statistical function without receiving recognition or compensation. Kenneth Miller, chief economist for Armour and Company, joined in the profuse tribute to the agency for the signal contribution it was making to the vital industry of meat packing. The inspectors continued to report the data, though grudgingly.

I cite this instance not only as an illustration of the nonmethodical origin of many data but to indicate how "consumption" was viewed. The data were the carcass weight of beef and lamb and product weight of pork going through processing channels. No correction was made for losses at any later stage. Then and to this day, to a very considerable extent, wholesale-level bias entered into data on disappearance of food products.

To complete my philosophical commentary on how statistical series came into being, the sequence very often has been that some program administrator needed new numbers. His statisticians scrambled to find whatever were available and engaged in some resourceful interpolating for those that were not. If the data proved truly useful their compilation was eventually assigned to a specialized agency, where corrections and refinements became attached. A fully clothed respectable statistical series then became a part of our data fund.

DATA FOR PRICE ANALYSIS

During the 1930's the commodity data for which program managers begged were those lending to statistical price analysis. Henry Schultz and Henry Moore were savants to whom Mordecai Ezekiel and Louis Bean gave allegiance. Price-determining forces were examined for a large collection of agricultural products. The quantity variable often was production or even total supply, rather than disappearance. The inadequacy of good distribution data was not regretted too much.

THE 1938 AGRICULTURAL LAW

I turn now to the writing of the Agricultural Adjustment Act of 1938. My chief, O. V. Wells, had a major hand in drafting the language of the law. In the previous 5 years a few persons had got the ear and conscience of Secretary of Agriculture Henry Wallace, telling him that the interests of consumers ought to be taken into account in designing and administering farm programs. Secretary Wallace was basically sympathetic but nearly impotent; however, in the 1938 act, language was inserted declaring a concern for protecting the supply of food for consumers. The act contained in its declaration of policy an injunction to assist consumers to obtain an adequate and steady supply of agricultural commodities at fair prices. Language in section 304 declared that nothing should be done to discourage producing supplies of food sufficient to maintain normal domestic human consumption as determined by the Secretary from records in the years 1920 to 1929, taking into account current trends in consumption and, significantly, the availability of substitutes. The years of the 1920's were a wise choice because the poorer nutrition of the 1930's, plagued by depression and drought, was thereby excluded.

Thereupon began a scramble for data on which to build credible food disappearance and consumption estimates. The first step was clerical. It was to print tabular cards on which supply and distribution data for the various farm commodities could be compiled. The cards had to have many columns. The physical ability to write and read numbers written in miniature longhand was virtually a requirement of employment in Mr. Wells' unit.

It would be a gold star on our national history if we could say that thereafter nutrition became an active ingredient in national farm policy. It did not. One reason, however, is that production outran markets so consistently that adequacy of food as such was not a serious issue.

Another consideration, however, came on the scene at about the same time. It was the proposal to distribute food to lower-income families. Once again the needs of a program, or potential program, were parent to the statistical progeny. In this case, however, a person of outstanding intellectuality was the sponsor. He was Frederick V. Waugh. His instincts were both humanitarian and economic. He turned the emphasis from national aggregates on food distribution to stratified data. He sought to apply Engel's law about food buying by income class. Demands grew to compile data on food consumption by regional and ethnic groups but especially by family income. The program involved was the new Food Stamp Plan, which was seen as a way both to improve the diets of low-income families and increase the total demand for farm products.

A few crude estimates began to appear as to the nutritional adequacy of householders' diets. An interesting offshoot were several studies, one by George Stigler, showing how cheaply a family could obtain adequate nutrition. The menu might be plain and dreary but it would have the minimum necessary nutrients.

Even the crudest nutritional analyses implicitly required estimates of waste in distribution of food. As I remember, the waste factor data were extremely poor. Again, getting hold of any kind of estimates required ingenuity more than technical ability.

All economists working on those studies were aware of another pitfall, namely, the meaning of "measures of central tendency." We might demonstrate that families of four with an income of $1,500 (in the valuable dollars of those days) would "consume" a quantity of protein or riboflavin equal to the minimum requirement. Obviously, approximately half would exceed the figure and half would fall short. The skewness of the distribution remained, as I recall, totally unknown. Even if the average exceeded the minimum by 20 percent, many of us suspected underconsumption by a considerable fraction of the families. We had almost no reliable estimates of skewness.

Of course, then as now, there were debates on just what figures best represented minimum nutritional requirements. But that is another subject.

HOUSEHOLD FOOD CONSUMPTION SURVEYS

It would be an injustice to fail to note the variety of statistical studies that had some incidental bearing on food consumption. Almost invariably the compilations had a purpose other than to indicate food consumption. The Census of Business gets expenditure data in its retail trade censuses. The Bureau of Labor Statistics has long assembled data on expenditure patterns for urban worker families as a source of weights for their consumer price indexes. For that matter, the U.S. Department of Agriculture has surveyed farm families for a similar purpose, namely, to update weight formulae for the "prices paid" index. More noteworthy are the decennial nationwide Household Food Consumption Surveys that began, as I remember, in 1955.

FOOD DIARIES

Probably the most complete data obtainable on families' spending for food are those derived from continuous diaries. I am most familiar with a Michigan State University diary study that continued for a number of years and with a Georgia Experiment Station diary enterprise that I believe to have been reinstigated. I regret to admit that I do not know to what extent the data so obtained have been exploited for appraisals of nutritional adequacy.

PREOCCUPATION WITH WHOLESALE DISTRIBUTION DATA

In this brief introduction I do not come close to doing justice to the virtual profusion of what I call bits and pieces studies relating to food distribution.

As a selected example, while writing these notes I came across Marketing Research Report No. 1017 of the Agricultural Research Service of USDA. (The agency has since been renamed.) It is titled *Marketing Losses of Selected Fruits and Vegetables*. I do not know whether Marketing Research Reports truly had reached the number of 1,017 by 1975 (the date of the study), but in any case a scanning of those reports would reveal lots of bits and pieces bearing in some way on quantification of food distribution.

The USDA deserves credit, in my opinion, for the great amount of work it has done. But I add quickly, and negatively, that the focus has almost always been on wholesale distribution; and this in turn is explained by preoccupation with assessing price-making influences. Often, the needs of operating programs have been paramount. Marketing orders, for example, are in force for fluid milk and well over 50 fruits, vegetables, and tree nuts. All these are statistically voracious.

Manifestly, the wholesale-level orientation implies a similar bias toward the original farm product identification. In distribution data it is easiest to trace through a product such as eggs, particularly if we do not worry too much about stratification of consumption. That is to say, an egg is an egg irrespective of whether it is eaten fried, scrambled, or part of a cake. But if aggregate consumption data are not sufficient and consumption data by classes are sought, we encounter the problem that the various groups of the population do not eat their eggs in the same ratios of fresh versus ingredients of processed foods.

The greater the amount of processing, the less meaningful are data expressed in the terms of the farm-identified commodity. This point is so clear, and its implications so complicating, that I need not develop it further. Dr. Van Meir and others on the 2-day program will clarify this problem, I am sure.

INSTITUTIONAL FOOD CONSUMPTION

I have left until last the topic of institutional food consumption. It has always been left until last. Only in fairly recent times have major projects been undertaken to assemble data on mass or institutional food programs in all their mazelike complexity. In a sense the wholesale bias has continued prominent.

I have not had occasion to dig into the institutional food issue in any depth. Persons working on this NRC project on food consumption patterns will doubtless do so.

My hunch is that the significance of institutional food services is not minor. Questions can be so simple such as whether noningestion is greater in institutional or household food consumption. My guess is that the ingestion ratio is highest in fast food services.

My attention has been directed recently to energy utilization in food distribution and preparation; and here the hypothesis is that institutional services can be energy conserving—except that the fast food business is energy-wasteful because of its profligate packaging.

REID, BURK, STIEBLING, AND OMAR KHAYAM

I caption my final remarks with the names Reid, Burk, Stiebling, and Omar Khayam. I am not sure what individuals most deserve gold medals for developing both data and awareness on food consumption. I know that in the U.S. Department of Agriculture all have had to fight for attention with the political figures who dole out dollars for CCC loans, P.L. 480 foreign food aid, and such. My hazy memory tells me that Jean Mayer was preceded long ago by a man named Henry Sherman. With regard to statistical data my mental association brings forth the names of Margaret Reid and Marguerite Burk; and the underrecognized advocate of giving nutrition more prominence in the design of farm programs was that grand lady, Hazel Stiebling. She was head of home economics in USDA. But my favorite citation in this connection is from Omar Khayam. He said he was no great guy; he was only trying to reduce the year to better reckoning. Perhaps we ought to award a few plaudits to those who now and henceforth try to reduce food distribution data to better reckoning. I personally applaud all those who will join the National Research Council in doing so. All I can add is that they will find a mixture of a wealth of bits and pieces, and gaping holes; and fitting the pieces together will prove to be an enormous jigsaw puzzle—but an interesting and worthwhile one.

Measurement and Forecasting of Food Consumption by USDA

ALDEN C. MANCHESTER *and*
KENNETH R. FARRELL

INTRODUCTION

In the federal government, responsibility for measuring and forecasting food consumption is in the Economics, Statistics, and Cooperatives Service (ESCS) of the Department of Agriculture. Consumption is an integral part of measurement and forecasting for food and agriculture, including production, stocks, international trade, and prices.

This paper discusses the system in which measures of per capita food consumption are developed, the sources and quality of the data used, and some of the uses of the data. It also considers data on food expenditures and some of its uses. It concludes with a discussion of the known deficiencies of the data base and possible steps to deal with the gaps.

THE SYSTEM FOR MEASURING CONSUMPTION

The basic concept is of a commodity flow data system (Figure 1). Agricultural products are produced on U.S. farms, caught by U.S. fishermen, or imported from abroad. Most move to manufacturing plants for processing and/or preservation. Then they move through the distribution system to retail stores or eating places and to consumers.

The USDA system measures all food in the commercial system. Farm home production of foods except vegetables also is measured. Rough estimates are made of farm garden vegetables and of nonfarm home production.

Food consumption is measured at the national aggregate level for 260 foods (see Appendix to this paper). There is no breakdown between food used at home and that used in restaurants and other away-from-home outlets. The use of supplements (vitamins, stabilizers, etc.) is not measured.

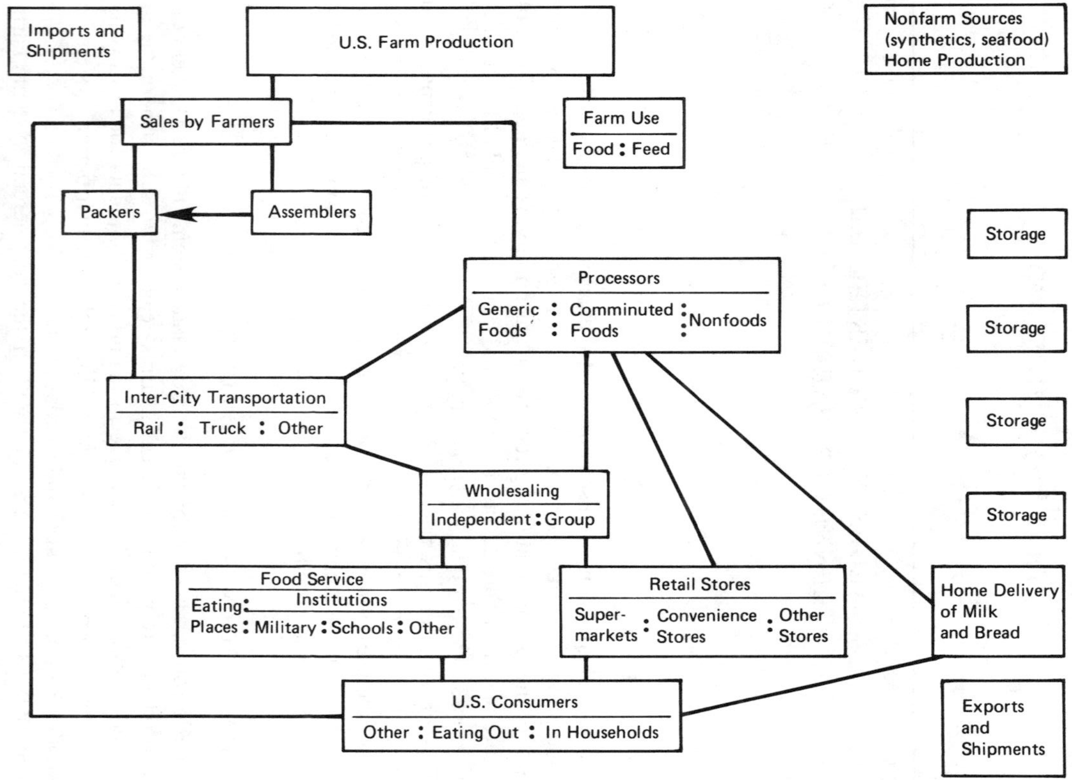

FIGURE 1 Commodity data system.

The basic tool is a supply and utilization balance sheet for each commodity (Table 1). Supply of each food consists of beginning stocks, production, imports, and in-shipments from territories (mostly Puerto Rico). Utilization consists of exports, shipments to territories, government purchases for military use and export, nonfood use, food use, and ending stocks. The availability of data is such that civilian food use is calculated as a residual after other measured uses are deducted from the total supply. Thus, it is often called disappearance.

Estimates of consumption (disappearance) are prepared at two levels for each commodity. The basic measurement is at the primary distribution level, which is dictated for each commodity by the structure of the marketing system and the availability of data. For some, it is at the farm gate. For most commodities which are processed, it is at the processing or manufacturing plant. Once the primary level of distribution has been selected, quantities of all other components in the balance sheet for that commodity are converted to the primary weight basis using appropriate conversion factors. For example, the primary distribution level for red meat is the slaughter plant, so all quantities are converted to carcass weight.

Most users of USDA consumption data are accustomed to the retail weight figures, which translate from primary distribution weight to retail weight by means of conversion factors that allow for subsequent processing and losses in the distribution system. Fresh beef, for instance, loses 26 percent of its weight from carcass to retail cuts.

For some uses, a more desirable basis of computation is edible weight. We have calculated per capita consumption on that basis for special articles (Manchester, 1977). That calculation avoids the problems that arise particularly because of the shift from fresh to processed products such as fruits and vegetables. We are developing such additional consumption series as an adjunct to those using primary distribution weight and retail weight.

The ideal system for nutritional analysis and many other uses would be one that measured actual ingestion of foods. No data are available to make such estimates for the U.S. population. While it seems highly unlikely that such data will ever become available except from carefully controlled laboratory tests, it may be possible to move closer to actual consumption. For example, the Market Research Corporation of America has conducted menu surveys that record foods actually served and those present. Such data give no assurance that the food was consumed by all present. And, of course, no attempt is made to measure quantity for each individual.

THE DATA—SOURCES AND QUALITY

The supply and utilization data system for food products is entirely dependent upon data that are collected for other purposes. No funds have ever

TABLE 1 Total Fats and Oils (Including Fat Content of Butter): Supply, Disposition, and Utilization, United States, 1963–76 (in millions of pounds)

	Supply			Disposition		
Year	Production from Domestic Materials[a]	Imports and Production from Imported Materials	Stocks, Jan. 1	Total	Exports[a, b]	Domestic Disappearance
1963	19,338	1,104	3,193	23,635	6,551	13,584
1964	20,672	1,131	3,599	25,402	8,211	14,368
1965	20,532	1,189	2,721	24,442	7,481	14,538
1966	21,013	1,359	2,445	24,817	6,725	15,312
1967	21,004	1,316	2,794	25,114	7,248	15,145
1968	21,496	1,398	2,668	25,562	7,354	15,698
1969	22,431	1,411	2,405	26,247	7,613	16,393
1970	25,012	1,363	2,286	28,661	10,150	16,119
1971	25,426	1,204	2,392	29,022	10,709	15,770
1972	25,347	1,459	2,543	29,349	10,465	16,340
1973	24,586	1,487	2,544	28,617	10,482	16,230
1974	26,824	1,389	1,905	30,118	11,768	16,374
1975	23,609	2,203	1,976	27,788	9,592	16,115
1976[d]	27,655	2,422	2,081	32,158	11,579	17,496

Utilization (Not Adjusted for Trade and Change in Stocks of Shortening, Margarine, Soap, and Secondaries)

	Food Uses						Nonfood Uses			
Year	Butter (Fat Content)	Lard (Direct)	Short-ening	Mar-garine	Other	Total	Soap[c]	Drying Oil Products	Other Indus-trial	Total
1963	1,083	1,191	2,611	1,450	2,470	8,805	797	879	3,252	4,928
1964	1,098	1,194	2,693	1,500	2,820	9,305	803	902	3,404	5,109
1965	1,040	1,226	2,768	1,534	2,949	9,517	746	909	3,347	5,002
1966	911	1,076	3,190	1,710	2,915	9,802	731	923	3,842	5,496
1967	887	1,056	3,243	1,703	3,012	9,901	718	859	3,855	5,432
1968	957	1,108	3,326	1,720	3,149	10,260	703	868	3,846	5,417
1969	908	1,012	3,505	1,744	3,620	10,789	706	738	4,169	5,613
1970	890	940	3,556	1,787	3,635	10,808	759	604	3,778	5,141
1971	860	881	3,490	1,811	3,720	10,762	745	631	3,724	5,100
1972	837	787	3,698	1,864	4,102	11,288	811	570	3,925	5,305
1973	812	705	3,614	1,884	4,322	11,337	728	686	3,743	5,153
1974	776	681	3,622	1,891	4,271	11,241	787	563	4,102	5,451
1975	819	632	3,666	1,907	4,298	11,322	808	429	3,778	5,015
1976[d]	762	568	3,861	2,069	4,688	11,948	944	547	4,240	5,731

[a] Includes oil equivalent of cottonseed, soybeans, peanuts, and flaxseed exported for crushing abroad.
[b] Includes commercial exports, voluntary or civilian relief, re-exports, and shipments to U.S. territories.
[c] Excludes an estimate of oil equivalent of soap used in synthetic rubber. This use is included in "Other Industrial."
[d] Preliminary.

been available to obtain data specifically on food consumption over time. Periodic surveys of food consumption or expenditures do provide useful checks. (For a detailed comparison of the disappearance data with Household Food Consumption Survey data, see LeBovit, 1968).

Data on farm production and stocks come primarily from the statistics program of ESCS. The ESCS statistics program also provides information on the uses of some products and the production of manufactured dairy products. Data on production of other processed products are obtained from other government and private sources, including *Current Industrial Reports* of the Bureau of the Census (for flour and fats and oils) and sugar utilization from the Agricultural Marketing Service. Where comprehensive data are available from trade associations, such as the National Food Processors Association, they are used.

Foreign trade data are compiled by the Bureau of the Census from Customs Service reports. Military use is reported by the Department of Defense for products procured through the central procurement system. Local procurement is estimated by USDA, primarily for milk and bread. Other data are used where available. A much more detailed account of the methods used and data sources is provided in *Major Statistical Series of the U.S. Department of Agriculture, How They Are Constructed and Used, Vol. 5: Consumption and Utilization of Agricultural Products,* U.S. Department of Agriculture, *Agriculture Handbook* No. 365, April 1972.

Major gaps exist because of the dependence on data collected for other purposes than measuring food consumption. A principal problem area is the measurement of food produced and consumed outside the commercial system—farm and nonfarm gardens, sport fish, and game. Survey data—such as the Household Food Consumption Survey (now the Nationwide Food Consumption Survey), which provides data once every 10–12 years—is now the principal source of such data. The difficulty is in developing satisfactory methods for making annual estimates with such data. In the last few years, ESCS has obtained better data on the number and size of home gardens through annual consumer surveys. When the results of the 1977–78 Nationwide Food Consumption Survey become available, we should be able to make reasonably good estimates for the years since the last survey in 1965–66. In terms of aggregate food consumption, gardens are fairly minor, accounting for only a few percent of total food. But, for some individual commodities of nutritional importance, they are far from trivial. In 1965–66, for example, home garden tomatoes accounted for 23 percent of all fresh tomatoes consumed at home.

Sport fish are similarly important, accounting for over half of all fish consumed in 1965–66. We have developed annual estimates of consumption of sport fish using the number of fishing licenses as a mover from the base provided by the 1965–66 survey. Again, the 1977–78 survey will provide a check on the reasonableness of these estimates.

Game animals are not a major source of meat, compared to that from farm production, although they contribute about as much to the diet as game fish. They are estimated similarly.

The other major problem area is also a result of the dearth of data. Most of the available current data are concentrated near the farm and primary processing levels. There are little or no data available for many further-processed products, especially comminuted or fabricated products such as bread, other bakery products, and soup. In short, relatively good data exist for the ingredients but not for many final products. Some of the firms represented at this workshop have data in more commodity detail for portions of the food market. No one has a data set with both the commodity detail we would all like to have and the detail by type of outlet.

NUTRITIVE VALUE OF THE FOOD SUPPLY

The Consumer and Food Economics Institute of the Science and Education Administration, USDA, utilizes the per capita consumption figures derived by ESCS to compute the nutritive value of the U.S. food supply for energy and 11 nutrients. The series shows trends in supplies of major nutrients that are related to changing food use patterns—the net effect in terms of nutrients of decreases in consumption of some foods and increases in others.

To obtain estimates of the nutritive value of the food supply, quantities of food consumed per capita per year are multiplied by the appropriate food composition values. Most of the composition values are from *Agriculture Handbook* No. 8 (Watt *et al.*, 1963) and its successors. No deduction is made for loss or waste of food in households or for destruction or loss of nutrients in the preparation of food.

Like all time series, regardless of what is being measured, the data are more useful as indicators of change over time than of absolute levels at any one time. In other words, this series provides an indication of whether or not Americans on the average are improving their diets over time. It is not a measure of nutritional adequacy.

EXPENDITURES

In 1978, ESCS introduced a new data series on *total* expenditures for food in the United States (Manchester, 1978; Manchester and King, 1979). Such a series has never been available before. The Department of Commerce, in the National Income and Product Accounts, has for many years estimated personal consumption expenditures for food, but this series intentionally excludes foods not paid for directly by individuals—i.e., meals on business expense accounts and in hospitals and institutions. The new series differentiates between food for use at home and that purchased in restaurants and furnished in hospitals and institutions. With appropriate adjustments for differences in price levels—which have been made—one can quantify the proportion of all food eaten at home, in public eating places, and elsewhere.

The new series is based on Bureau of the Census data on retail sales by type of establishment—grocery stores, drug stores, restaurants, etc.—where available. These account for the biggest part of the basic data in the system. Thus, it is possible to estimate total food expenditures for regions and states, an advantage for many forms of economic analysis and probably also for analyses of food programs and other nutrition-related problems.

The new series on total food expenditures is consistent with the quantity figures supplied by the consumption data discussed in the preceding sections. The coverage of both series is all food and the basic equation—price × quantity = value—holds. In other words, consumption (quantity) times price equals expenditures, when retail store prices are used both in the price variable and in expenditures.

FORECASTING

Basically, forecasting is an extension into the future of the system previously described. The obvious difference is that we are no longer attempting to measure what has happened but are attempting to indicate what is most likely to happen next month or next year, given what we know about the current and prospective situation and the economic relationships involved. The basis is forecasts of production, exports, imports, and changes in stocks. These are analyzed in terms of their effects on prices and the effects of those prices on consumer willingness to purchase.

DETERMINANTS OF CONSUMPTION AND DEMAND

In the short run, it is a truism that what is produced is consumed; in economists' terms, that supply equals demand. The great equilibrator is price. When supplies go up, price goes down and consumers buy and consume more. Conversely, smaller supplies bring higher prices and smaller purchases. Demand for food in the aggregate is inelastic—i.e., not very responsive to price changes. Demand for individual foods is more elastic. Over time, rising incomes increase expenditures on more expensive foods. Thus, short-period changes in consumption reflect mostly changes in supply rather than changes in consumer tastes or wants. The demand schedule, in economists' terms, may not have changed at all, although—because of larger supplies and lower prices—consumption may be much larger than it was in a previous year.

Sources of Change, 1954–76

Analysis of the sources of changes in food expenditures between 1954—the first year of the ESCS Total Food Expenditure series—and 1976 provides a background for consideration of the factors affecting food expenditures and consumption.

Food expenditures increased from $366 per person in 1954 to $443 in 1965 and $939 in 1976 (Table 2). Food-at-home expenditures more than doubled. Food away-from-home more than tripled. The biggest increase was in expenditures for meals and snacks in public eating places—up four times.

Prices doubled in grocery stores (Table 3) and rose substantially more in restaurants. Quantities consumed (in pounds) went down a bit, although the price-weighted per capita food consumption index rose 10 percent, reflecting the shift to higher-valued foods, especially beef. Over the same 22-year period, disposable income per capita rose 250 percent—much more than the increases in food expenditures.

A combination of consumption and expenditures data allows us to sort out the components of change. Out of a $573 increase in per capita food expenditures from 1954 to 1976, the biggest share was due to price change, $416 (73 percent) (Table 4). The shift in outlets—primarily from home to away-from-home—increased per capita food expenditures by $62 (11 percent), while changes in quantities accounted for $34 (6 percent), and shifts between foods for $61 (10 percent) per person.

Demographic factors—change in household size and in the age–sex distribution—would have brought about an increase of about $28 per person over this period, even if nothing else had changed.

TABLE 2 Food Expenditures Per Capita, 1954, 1965, and 1976 (in dollars per person)

	1954	1965	1976
Food at home:			
Purchased	252	293	584
Home-produced and donations	22	18	32
TOTAL	274	311	616
Food away-from-home			
Public eating places	59	93	246
Limited clientele	15	20	32
Meals furnished	18	19	45
TOTAL	92	132	323
All food	366	443	939

TABLE 3 Factors Affecting Food Expenditures, 1954, 1965, and 1976

	1954	1965	1976
Consumer price indexes for food:			
Grocery store prices	100	111	209
Restaurant prices	100	130	265
Farm value	100	103	185
Wholesale prices	100	107	199
Per capita food consumption:			
Index	100	101	110
Pounds	100	97	99
Disposable income per capita:			
Current dollars	1,574	2,430	5,511
Index	100	154	300

TABLE 4 Sources of Change in Food Expenditures Per Capita from 1954 to 1965 and 1976 (in dollars)

	Change from 1954 to:	
	1965	1976
Change due to:		
Shift in outlets	+19	+ 62
Changes in prices	+52	+416
Changes in quantities	+ 2	+ 34
Shifts among food groups	− 1	+ 55
Shifts among foods within food groups	+ 5	+ 6
TOTAL CHANGES	+77	+573

Highly Processed Foods

The available data can be used to shed additional light on the changes in food consumption patterns. As an example, let's consider the consumption of highly processed foods.

For this analysis, data provided annually by *Supermarketing Magazine*, which give detail for products in final form as they appear in the retail store or enter the restaurant kitchen, are deflated by appropriate price indexes so that each year is in effect calculated at 1971 prices (Manchester, 1977a,b) (Table 5). Thus, approximations of *change* in quantities—not measures of actual quantity—are obtained.

The strongest impression is stability. Products that are unchanged from the raw state except for having been cleaned, slaughtered, dressed, or preserved—fresh meat, poultry, milk, eggs, fresh and processed fruits, and vegetables—accounted for two-thirds of the value of all food in each of the

TABLE 5 Food Consumption by Degree of Processing, 1952, 1971, and 1975 (percent[a])

Item	1952	1971	1975
Products unchanged from raw state except that they are:			
Cleaned, slaughtered, or dressed	36.6	38.7	39.8
Preserved	30.4	28.8	27.3
SUBTOTAL	67.0	67.5	67.1
Manufactured products:			
Derived mainly from a single raw product	10.5	10.1	11.0
Combine ingredients	22.5	22.4	21.9
SUBTOTAL	33.0	32.5	32.9
TOTAL	100.0	100.0	100.0

[a] Percent of value of total domestic food consumption at 1971 retail store prices.

SOURCE: Basic data from *Supermarketing Magazine*. Price level adjustments and classification by ESCS.

years; and manufactured products—those that combine a number of ingredients—represented virtually the same share of the value in 1952 and 1971 and then dropped 0.5 percentage points between 1971 and 1975. Thus, it would appear that the much-touted turnaway from highly processed products by consumers when prices rose rapidly in 1973 and 1974 did occur, although on a fairly modest scale.

Bigger shifts occurred between products that are preserved by canning, freezing, heating, or drying than those that are merely cleaned, slaughtered, or dressed. Here the changes between 1952 and 1971 toward less preservation continued in the same direction to 1975.

DATA GAPS

Because the ESCS food consumption data system is dependent upon the availability of data collected for other purposes, there are major data gaps. The most serious occur as we get nearer to the consumer in the food chain.

Farm production is well covered by an increasingly sophisticated statistical system. Reduction in the coverage of production caused by budget constraints has created problems in a few areas—notably fresh vegetables. Production of some minor vegetables is no longer reported annually, nor is the production of major vegetables in minor states. This makes very little difference in the total farm picture or in total food consumption, but may be significant for monitoring the consumption of nutrients for which these vegetables are important sources.

Imports and exports are covered almost completely as a by-product of customs service activity.

Manufacture of primary products is now covered relatively well by a combination of agencies. Meat slaughter and dairy product production is reported by USDA. Fats and oils, confectionery, and flour are reported by the Bureau of the Census in their Current Industrial Reports. The pack of canned and frozen fruits and vegetables are covered by the National Food Processors Association and the Frozen Food Institute.

Manufacture of secondary products is covered much less completely. The production of products that combine a number of food ingredients is most commonly reported only by the Census of Manufactures every 5 years. Products in this category include canned and frozen prepared foods; jams, jellies, and preserves; baked goods, including bread; breakfast cereals; baby foods; condiments and sauces; and ready-to-mix desserts.

Soups are not reported at all, even in the Census, because of the dominance of one company. The problem of disclosing the operations of that company led to a decision by the Bureau of the Census not to report all information for soup. The last complete statistics for soup are for 1946.

Manufacture at retail is not reported at all. The largest gap here is for retail bakeries. We know how much flour is produced monthly. We know how it is used in manufacturing bakeries and other plants (e.g., breakfast cereals) 1 year in 5. We can only infer the amount of flour going into retail bakeries from the unaccounted-for use of bulk flour, assuming that smaller packages are all used in households. What the retail baker makes from that flour we have no way of knowing at any time. With retail bakeries making annual sales of $2 billion, it is not insignificant. And these sales do not include in-store bakeries in supermarkets.

Away-from-home food consumption has been studied only once, in 1969 (Van Dress and Freund, 1968, 1971, 1972a, 1972b), although the Institutional Food Manufacturers Association is now updating the 1969 survey. We are now purchasing data from National Diary Panel, Inc., based on a quarterly diary from a sample of households which provides expenditure data on away-from-home purchases of food and some limited data on the foods purchased, primarily for the main course.

Household food purchases are reported regularly by a number of commercial survey organizations, but no one covers all foods. A number of firms operate panels that report purchases of selected foods on a regular basis. The long-time operator in this field is the Market Research Corporation of America. The foods covered are primarily packaged items, because those are the ones their clients are interested in.

For a number of years, the Economic Research Service and now the Economics, Statistics, and Cooperatives Service have been interested in obtaining data from a national consumer panel that reports purchases of all foods on a regular basis. Such a panel, using a national probability sample of adequate size, would give us information on the use of foods in the household by various income and family size groups, food stamp recipients, the poor, families with and without children, and many other groups. The main obstacle is money. Such a panel would be expensive.

Such panels for all foods have been operated by universities in several cities in the past. The Georgia Experiment Station is currently operating a small panel in Griffin, Ga.

The Bureau of Labor Statistics (BLS) has plans to start a Continuing Consumer Expenditures Survey. It is planned to utilize a 2-week diary each quarter for food purchases, with the sample of households remaining in the survey for probably five quarters and a portion rotating each quarter. While the diary will provide space for recording quantities of food as well as expenditures, BLS experience in the past has been that only a portion of panel members actually record quantity data. Present plans provide for a delay of approximately a year between data collection and publication.

For several years, ESCS attempted to establish a probability panel of retailers and wholesalers who would report current movement of all foods into retail stores. This is similar to Selling Areas Marketing, Inc., but would cover all foods, including perishable items and those delivered directly to the retail store and not moving through the warehouse. This effort was initiated because of an interest in retail prices and marketing margins, but it would yield substantial information on food sales by retail stores. Unfortunately, we have been unable to obtain cooperation from the retailers, because of their concern over possible disclosure of financial data.

Stocks

Per capita consumption data are now available annually for all foods and quarterly for animal products. The major gap preventing compilation of quarterly figures for crop products is the lack of stocks data on a quarterly basis, so we can tell how much of a given product has moved into consumption from the current season's pack. We are working on methods of overcoming this problem short of expensive additional data collection.

Expenditures

A number of items in the expenditures series are estimated by less-than-satisfactory methods. These include food use in colleges and universities, hospitals, and institutions. Home food production is also measured poorly, both for quantities and value.

SUMMARY

ESCS compiles national food consumption statistics for 260 different foods and food expenditure statistics covering all food. The basic data that enter these calculations are largely a by-product of other interests. No funds are or have been available to USDA specifically to obtain food consumption or expenditure statistics on a continuing basis.

There are major gaps in these statistics once we leave the farm or first manufacture level. Thus, consumption of each food is measured at the last level for which data obtained for other purposes are available. Flour consumption is measured, not bakery and cereal products, for example. Filling these gaps will be an expensive process, but it needs to be done.

We badly need comprehensive data on consumption or, at the minimum, purchases by households of food both for use in the home and away from home. With such data, the system can be closed—measuring production or manufacture at each level where it occurs and sales to the final consumer at the other end.

A consumer panel would provide data for different types of households on food purchases for home use and some information on away-from-home consumption, although not in the same detail as for that used at home. This would improve the national consumption statistics and have the additional benefit of permitting the analysis of consumption by individual households of different size and composition, income levels, and other characteristics. With a large enough sample, such data would also permit separation of food stamp recipients from other households of similar characteristics who were not participating.

Detailed data on food store sales (or receipts) of individual goods would be almost as useful as data from a consumer panel in many ways. It would provide better detail on individual products than it is possible to obtain from households. It would not, of course, be helpful in analysis of consumption or purchases by different types of households.

The BLS Continuing Consumer Expenditures Survey will be helpful, although it is probably not realistic to expect high-quality data, if any, on the quantities of individual foods purchased. Its other chief drawback, from our point of view, is the 1-year time lag between collection and publication.

REFERENCES

LeBovit, Corinne. 1968. U.S. food consumption: Annual disappearance and household survey data. Natl. Food Sit., November 1968, pp. 32–41.

Manchester, Alden C. 1977a. Are highly processed foods taking over the market? Natl. Food Sit., March 1977, p. 34.

Manchester, Alden C. 1977b. Eating more vegetables. Natl. Food Sit., March 1977, pp. 34–35.

Manchester, Alden C. 1978. Total food expenditures—A new series. Natl. Food Rev., April 1978, pp. 16–17.

Manchester, Alden C., and Richard A. King. 1979. U.S. food expenditures, 1954–78: New measures at point of sales and by type of purchaser. Econ. Res. Rep. Agric. Econ. Rep. No. 431, August 1979. 26 pp.

Van Dress, Michael G., and William H. Freund. 1968. The food service industry: Its structure and characteristics, 1966. U.S. Econ. Res. Serv. Stat. Bull. No. 416, February 1968. 370 pp.

Van Dress, Michael G., and William H. Freund. 1971. The food service industry: Type, quantity, and value of foods used. U.S. Econ. Res. Serv. Stat. Bull. No. 476, November 1971. 451 pp.

Van Dress, Michael G., and William H. Freund. 1972a. Separate eating places: Type, quantity and value of foods used. U.S. Econ. Res. Serv. Stat. Bull. No. 487, June 1972. 223 pp.

Van Dress, Michael G., and William H. Freund. 1972b. The market for food consumed away from home: Dollar value statistics. U.S. Econ. Res. Serv. Stat. Bull. No. 491, September 1972. 105 pp.

Watt, Bernice K., Annabel L. Merrill, *et al.* 1963. Composition of foods—Raw, processed, prepared. U.S. Agric. Res. Serv. Agric. Handb. No. 8, Rev., December 1963. 190 pp.

APPENDIX: FOOD COMMODITIES COVERED IN CONSUMPTION STATISTICS

	Primary Distribution Level
MEAT	
Beef	Slaughter
Veal	Slaughter
Pork	Slaughter
Lamb	Slaughter
Edible offal (variety meats)	Slaughter
POULTRY	
Young chickens (broilers)	Slaughter
Other chickens	Slaughter
Turkey	Slaughter
EGGS	
Shell	Farm
Processed	Manufacture
DAIRY PRODUCTS	Manufacture
Fluid milk products:	
Whole milk	
Lowfat and skim milk	
Cream and half and half	
Sour cream products	
Yogurt	
Butter	

Cheese (16 varieties)
Cottage cheese
Nonfat dry milk
Evaporated milk
Condensed milk
Dried whole milk
Dried buttermilk
Ice cream
Sherbet
Ice milk
Mellorine
Water ices
Dry whey

FISH AND SEAFOOD (National Marine Fisheries Service)

	Edible Weight
Fresh and frozen:	
Salmon	
Other fish	
Shrimp	
Northern lobster	
Spiny lobster	
Oysters	
Clams	
Crabs	
Scallops	
Canned:	
Salmon	
Sardines (pilchards and herring)	
Tuna	
Shellfish	
Other	
Cured	

FRUITS	Fresh	Canned	Frozen	Dried	Chilled
Citrus:					
Oranges	x				
Tangelos	x				
Tangerines	x				
Lemons	x				
Limes	x				
Grapefruit	x				
Citrus sections		x			x
Citrus juice:					
Orange juice		x	x		x
Grapefruit juice		x	x		x
Citrus concentrate		x			
Blended orange and grapefruit juice		x	x		
Lemon and lime juice		x			
Tangerine juice		x	x		

	Fresh	Canned	Frozen	Dried	Chilled
Lemon juice			x		
Lemonade			x		
Limeade			x		
Noncitrus:					
Apples	x	x	x	x	
Apricots	x	x	x	x	
Avocados	x				
Bananas	x				
Bushberries	x	x	x		
Cherries	x	x	x		
Cranberries	x	x			
Figs	x	x		x	
Grapes	x		x		
Nectarines	x				
Peaches	x	x	x	x	
Pears	x	x		x	
Pineapple	x	x			
Papayas	x				
Plums and prunes	x	x		x	
Strawberries	x		x		
Miscellaneous fruit	x		x		
Salad and cocktail		x			
Olives		x			
Apple juice		x			
Grape juice		x			
Pineapple juice		x			
Prune juice		x			
Dates				x	
Raisins				x	

VEGETABLES	Fresh	Canned	Frozen	Dehydrated
Artichokes	x			
Asparagus	x	x	x	
Beans, lima		x	x	
Beans, snap (green)	x	x	x	
Broccoli	x		x	
Brussels sprouts			x	
Cabbage	x			
Carrots	x	x	x	
Kale	x			
Lettuce and escarole	x			
Peas, green	x	x	x	
Peppers	x			
Spinach	x	x	x	
Other vegetables	x	x	x	
Beets		x		
Cauliflower	x		x	
Celery	x			
Corn	x	x	x	

	Fresh	Canned	Frozen	Dehydrated
Cucumbers	x			
Eggplant	x			
Garlic	x			
Onions and shallots			x	x
Tomatoes	x	x		
Pumpkin and squash		x		
Catsup and chili sauce, tomato paste and sauce		x		
Tomato pulp and puree		x		
Tomato and other vegetable juices		x		
Pickles		x		
Sauerkraut		x		
Peas and carrots			x	
Southern greens			x	
Potatoes	x	x	x	x
Potato chips and shoestrings				x
Sweet potatoes	x	x		
MELONS				
Watermelons	x			
Cantaloupes, honeydew	x			
PEANUTS	Manufacture			
Peanut butter				
Salted peanuts				
Peanut candy				
Peanut butter sandwiches				
Unshelled peanuts				
FATS AND OILS	Manufacture			
Margarine				
Lard				
Shortening				
Cooking and salad oils				
Other edible (salad dressings, mayonnaise, etc.)				
BEANS, PEAS AND SOY PRODUCTS	Farm			
Dry edible beans				
Dry field peas				
Soya grits and flour				
CEREAL PRODUCTS	Manufacture			
Wheat flour:				
White and whole wheat				
Semolina and durum flour				
Wheat cereal				
Rye flour				
Rice				

Corn products:	
Flour and meal	
Cereal	
Starch	
Hominy and grits	
Oat food products	
Barley products	
SWEETENERS	Manufacture
Sugar, cane	
Sugar, beet	
Corn, dextrose (refined corn sugar)	
Honey	
Syrups:	
Corn, high fructose	
Corn, glucose	
Maple	
Sugar cane	
Sorgo	
Refiners	
Edible cane molasses	
Saccharin (sugar sweetener equivalent)	
CONFECTIONERY	Manufacture
COFFEE	Manufacture
Roasted	
Instant	
TEA	Imports
COCOA	Imports
SOFT DRINKS	Manufacture
TREE NUTS	Imports or production
Almonds	
Filberts	
Pecans	
Walnuts	
Macadamia	
Other tree nuts	
Coconut	
SPICES AND HERBS	Imports or production
Pepper	
Mustard seed	
Chili peppers	
Anise seed	

Caraway seed
Celery seed
Cinnamon
Cloves
Coriander seed
Cumin seed
Fennel seed
Ginger root
Mace
Nutmeg
Paprika
Pimento (Allspice)
Poppy seed
Sage
Sesame Seed
Turmeric
Vanilla beans
Other spices

Aggregate Measures of Food Consumption

Retail Weight of Food Consumed Per Capita The main purpose for developing a uniform measure for consumption at the retail level is to facilitate the development of the price-weighted index. However, these data are useful by themselves for measuring trends and shifts, especially at an unaggregated level of food groups. For example, the substitution within the fresh fruit or fresh vegetable categories can be reasonably identified with this measure. Shifts within the canned product categories can be accurately measured. The substitution of beef for pork on a poundage basis can be traced over time.

This measure of civilian per capita disappearance is computed from primary weight consumption data. For example, beef is measured on a carcass weight basis, a form in which it leaves the packing plant. A factor that reflects cutting loss, trim, and bones is applied to the carcass weight. The primary weight of fresh fruits and vegetables is a farm weight. Different factors are used to equate the farm weight to a retail weight basis.

A total food consumption measure in terms of total (retail-weight) pounds is published. This series has been quite stable at a little over 1,400 pounds in recent years. However, the total pounds consumed peaked out in 1945. The consumption of crop products by this measure has shown the most decline as consumers have shifted to more processed products.

Also, there may be some double counting in this series. Adjustments are made for sugar and butter. Sugar in canned fruits for example is included in the canned fruit total but subtracted from the sugar and other sweetener total.

Index of Per Capita Consumption The index of per capita food consumption is probably the best economic measure of the food consumed at the retail level. Pounds of food consumed on a retail weight basis are combined with retail store prices in a base period to measure annual or quarterly changes in food consumption. While the index primarily measures quantity changes, it also reflects shifts such as those from a low priced to a higher-priced food. This could indicate the shift from cereal products to animal products and the shift from fresh to processed forms.

The consumption data include the significant portion of food consumed away from home as well as food consumed on farms where produced. The shift to away from home is not reflected in the index.

This index can rise though the quantities consumed may be unchanged from year to year. For example, as family incomes rise, shifts to more expensive items such as chicken to beef would result in a higher index of consumption. This index has generally increased during the past decade as consumption has switched to higher-priced foods. It reached a record high in 1976 and has declined slightly during the past 2 years as red meat supplies have tapered off.

This index is published for 27 different groups, which include animal product and crop product categories.

A similar food use index is also available. It measures changes in domestic consumption at the farm level. Farm prices are used to weight the index and even the value of processed products is factored back to the farm level. This index has risen less than the per capita consumption index, since the shifts to more processed forms are washed out by the indexing procedure. However, shifts in the mix of food used would have an influence on the index.

Nutritive Value of Food Consumed The retail weight equivalent of food consumed is the basis for developing the nutrient values for food energy, protein, fat, carbohydrate, calcium, phosphorus, iron, magnesium, vitamin A, thiamin, riboflavin, niacin, vitamin B_6, vitamin B_{12}, and ascorbic acid. Quantities of food consumed are multiplied by appropriate food composition values. The information is published as nutrients available for per capita consumption per day and percentages of total nutrients contributed by 24 major food categories.

A. C. Nielsen Company Services

OLIVER S. CASTLE

The Nielsen Food Index (NFI) service is the comprehensive national service covering products sold through grocery stores in all 48 contiguous states. All data are projected to national and regional totals and shown separately by the 10 Nielsen geographic areas (Figure 1), by store type (chain grocery versus independents), and the latter by volume classifications (Table 1). Other divisions, such as client sales areas, are available as ordered.

Consumer sales and shares (Table 2) are reported bimonthly by brand and product group in dollars and by a physical measurement—either pounds, units, gallons, etc. Retail inventories and retailer purchases are reported in the same fashion.

Retail distribution, for each brand and size, provides a measure of the stores handling each brand and size and are computed in two ways. Store count distribution, as the name implies, reports on the actual number of stores handling a brand. All-commodity distribution is weighted by store dollar volume. As such this measure reflects the extent to which each major brand is exposed to all grocery activity based upon the total dollar sales of the stores handling the brand.

Measures of out-of-stock are also reported on a store count and all-commodity basis and are projected to national and regional areas. Out-of-stock when computed on an all-commodity basis reveals the relative importance of stores without the item or items in question on the date of audit, but handling the item during the 2-month period between audits.

Average retail prices are available for each brand, size, and type by area and nationally. These prices, keep in mind, are prices charged to consumers by retailers.

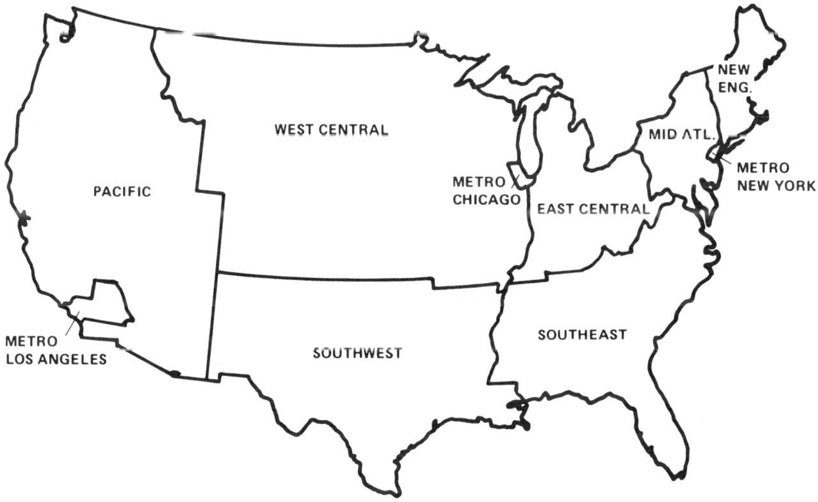

FIGURE 1 Nielsen territories.

We also produce sales influencing data based on observations in each sample store relative to special prices and in-store displays. All advertising that originates with the sample stores, including that of corporate chain stores, is also checked every audit period. These data are reported for each brand on an all-commodity basis nationally and by Nielsen territory.

The means are essentially some 650 full-time field representatives, 62 district managers and 8 regional managers. All field representatives are

TABLE 1 NFI Services

Data Breakdowns Available

Brand, Type, and Size	Territory	Client Areas		County Sizes	Store Types
Private	New England	1	10	Metro New York	Grocery
Label	Metro New York	2	11	Metro Chicago	Chains (4 or more stores)
Brands	Mid. Atlantic	3	12	Metro Los Angeles	Large—Over 500 M
	East Central	4	13	A Counties	annual sales
National	Metro Chicago	5	14	B Counties	Medium—under 500 M
and	West Central	6	15	C Counties	annual sales
regional	Southeast	7	16	D Counties	Independents
brands	Southwest	8	17		Large—Over 500 M
by name,	Metro Los Angeles	9	18		Medium—100-500 M
type, and	Pacific				Small—Under 100 M
size					

TABLE 2 NFI Services

Consumer sales and shares reported bimonthly in—
Dollars
By a Physical Measurement:
Units,
Pounds,
Gallons,
etc.

college educated, then trained from 6 to 9 months in Nielsen's field training school, and finally given several more months of training in the field with experienced field representatives selected for this purpose. The end result is a field staff that is unique in terms of caliber, training and size and one not duplicated by any other market research firm. This staff, supervised by district managers, enables Nielsen to handle a variety of complex projects in addition to the painstaking audits of the sample stores.

What then is the primary function of each member of the field staff relative to the distribution and sales of grocery items?

The field representatives' goals are to determine the movement of each and every grocery item by brand, size, and type in the product classes under audit and in the stores included in the sample (Table 3). The table is based on a bimonthly period, but monthly or weekly audits are performed in the same fashion.

TABLE 3 Principles of Nielsen Retail Index Auditing (''Alpha'' Brand of Dry Soup Mix in Super X Market)

	For June–July: Pkgs.	Value
Inventory		
May 30	114	
July 30	93	
Change	21	
Purchases		
From manufacturer (1 order)	12	\$ 3.72
From wholesalers (4 orders)	48	15.00
Total	60	\$18.72
Consumer sales		
Packages	81	
Price, per pkg.		\$ 0.39
Dollars, total		\$31.59
Adv. 1 2 3 4 5		
6 7 8 9		
Display X	Selling price 39¢	
	Special price 35¢	

In the example, the 114 units were the inventory the retailer had on hand at the end of the previous audit—the 93 units represent the current inventory. Total sales of the item during the period amounted to 81 units—a 21-unit change in inventory plus the purchases of 60 units during the period.

In addition, the brand was on display, as noted by the X, and had been advertised six separate times by the retailer during the past 60 days. The item was selling for 39¢ on the date of audit but had been advertised at the special price of 35¢ during the period. Since the auditor separates the inventory of each item on a reserve versus the selling area of the store, it is possible to show the percentage of the inventory which is visible to customers (i.e., selling area).

As you can see, the audit is simple in itself but to obtain the correct numbers—inventories, purchases, etc.—for every brand, size, and type in a giant supermarket, it becomes a complex and meticulous task—hence the careful screening of field personnel and extensive training and supervision.

Nielsen is currently auditing 152 food and beverage product classes, including frozen and refrigerated products. This includes a wide variety of packaged, nonperishable foods in cans, cartons, bottles, jars, etc.—primarily warehouse items. But Nielsen, by concentrating its efforts at the store or retail level, is able also to cover store–door delivered items. These include the great majority of soft drinks, crackers, cheese, and significant amounts of snack items and refrigerated and frozen foods that do not pass through either chain or wholesale warehouses. It further means that we can provide complete data on drop-shipments of any other packaged food products that are delivered directly from the manufacturer to the store and thus bypassing all warehouses.

There are many other standard grocery product groups—such as detergents, toilet soap, floor wax, paper towels, and so forth—that are not edible but have been handled in grocery stores for as long as these outlets have been in existence. This would add another 61 groups for a total of 213.

In addition to the national service, we also cover 38 major markets by using supplemental samples specifically designed for and projectable to the designated market. Each market includes the central city, the suburbs, and remaining television area. The areas are large enough to ensure that products in question are exposed to a broad range of people, demographically, and the close conformity to the television areas allows for measurement of television promotional activity.

The identical types of data produced for the national service are available, that is—consumer sales and shares, retail inventories, distribution, sales rates, etc., measured on both a dollar and physical basis. Figures 2 and 3 show two typical areas: Rochester, N.Y., and Miami–Ft. Lauderdale, Fla.

Table 4 lists the entire 38 markets. Combined, they account for 61.4 percent of the population and 62.3 percent of total grocery sales.

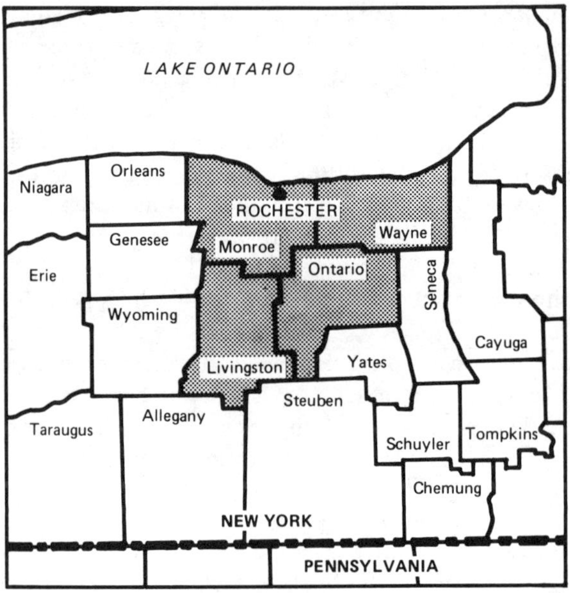

FIGURE 2 Rochester, N.Y.

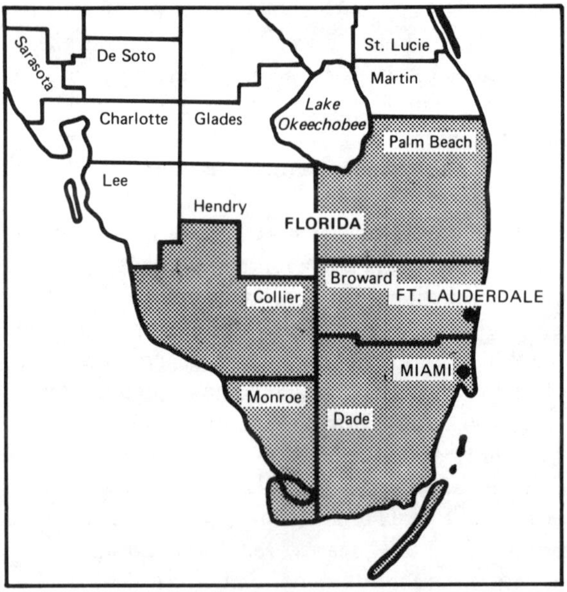

FIGURE 3 Miami–Ft. Lauderdale, Fla.

TABLE 4 Nielsen Major Markets

	Metro Areas	% of U.S. Population (Jan. 1, 1976)	% of U.S. Grocery Sales (1975)	% of U.S. Drug Sales (1975)
Areas with Populations Larger Than 2.0% of U.S.	New York	7.5	6.9	5.9
	Los Angeles	4.7	4.9	5.8
	Chicago	3.6	3.4	4.8
	Philadelphia	3.6	3.7	3.2
	Baltimore–Wash., D.C.	3.2	3.2	4.3
	Boston	3.2	3.2	2.8
	Detroit	2.9	3.1	3.7
	San Francisco–Oakland	2.3	2.6	3.2
	Cleveland	2.1	2.3	1.9
	Pittsburgh	2.0	1.8	1.7
Areas with Populations between 1.9% and 1.0% of U.S.	Dallas–Ft. Worth	1.5	1.6	1.6
	Miami–Ft. Lauderdale	1.4	1.8	1.9
	Minneapolis–St. Paul	1.4	1.3	1.2
	St. Louis	1.4	1.4	1.3
	Atlanta	1.3	1.4	1.3
	Cincinnati	1.3	1.2	1.1
	Houston	1.3	1.5	1.2
	Indianapolis	1.3	1.1	1.4
	Seattle–Tacoma	1.1	1.3	1.3
	Kansas City	1.0	0.9	0.9
	Memphis	1.0	0.9	0.7
	Milwaukee	1.0	0.9	0.8
	Portland	1.0	1.2	1.0
Areas with Populations under 1.0% of U.S.	Buffalo	0.9	0.9	0.9
	Denver	0.9	0.9	1.0
	Nashville	0.8	0.9	0.8
	Phoenix	0.8	0.9	0.9
	Sacramento–Stockton	0.8	0.9	1.2
	Birmingham–Anniston	0.7	0.7	0.6
	Charlotte	0.7	0.7	0.7
	Grand Rapids–Kalamazoo	0.7	0.8	0.6
	Louisville	0.7	0.6	0.6
	Albany–Schenectady–Troy	0.6	0.7	0.5
	Oklahoma City	0.6	0.6	0.5
	Omaha	0.6	0.5	0.6
	San Antonio	0.6	0.6	0.5
	Jacksonville	0.5	0.5	0.7
	Rochester	0.4	0.5	0.5
TOTAL MAJOR MARKET AREAS		61.4	62.3	63.6

NOTE: All population and household data are from *Sales and Marketing Management* magazine estimates and, unless otherwise stated, refer to the condition as of January 1, 1976. Store count and volume data are Nielsen estimates and refer to 1975.

Back in 1959, when the research and development of new products were becoming a way of life for large grocery manufacturers, the need for a data source that was both broad in scope, i.e., encompassing virtually all products sold through supermarkets and yet reliable enough to identify and evaluate growth opportunities in the grocery field became apparent.

To fill this need, we developed a new system of services called Nielsen Early Intelligence System (NEIS). The basic service in this system—Data Services—is based on a summary of warehouse-to-store shipments of all grocery items from a nationwide sample of 150 supermarkets and reported every 60 days. First, all packaged grocery items are merged into 600 logical product groups—but each individual brand within the group is reported separately by brand, size, type, flavor, etc. Some 430 product groups are edible foods, and the remaining 170 are assorted product categories such as detergents, soaps, health and beauty aids, and other general merchandise.

We originally thought the primary use, and perhaps sole use of Data Services, would be to identify and quickly appraise product areas of opportunity for manufacturers interested in developing new products and markets outside of their areas of interest. Even though the service was eminently successful in this regard, we soon discovered, as did our clients, that the data had additional uses or applications in a variety of other situations. Table 5 shows a sample report page from Data Services.

The product class used in the table is Canned Beef Stew. Note that the unit movement for the total market for October–November 1977 compared to the same period of 1976 reveals an increase of some 2,900 units or over 7 percent versus a dollar gain of about 8 percent.

Also provided are data for each brand of beef stew by size, type, flavor, etc. Note that Dinty Moore Beef Stew had a 1977 unit share of 48.7 percent of the total market, up four points from the previous year, and a 53.5 percent share of the dollars spent for beef stews. During this 1977 period, 99 percent of the sample stores purchased at least one size of the brand indicating wide distribution, and average unit movement for the brand was 12.7 cans per week.

These same data are provided in identical form for each and every brand in a product group—however many there are. Thus, it is readily apparent that the entire range of food products can be monitored in order to detect any major changes or shifts in consumer preferences or product innovations.

Table 6 provides a "shopping list" of the types of information our clients have obtained from Nielsen Early Intelligence Systems. As you can see, the real strength of this service is its ability to answer straightforward questions with direct answers relative to marketing trends in terms of prices, packages, types, etc.

Point three may need a moment's explanation. By "controlled brands"

TABLE 5 Nielsen Early Intelligence System Data Services—Directory Report P.C. #1221—Canned Beef Stew

				Total Units		Total Dollars		Stores Purch., %		Weekly Unit Movement	
Brand Description	Size	Case Pack	Avg. Unit Retail	O–N '76	O–N '77	O–N '76	O–N '77	'76	'77	'76	'77
Total Market				41,607	44,578	36,925	40,094				
Share of Market				100.0%	100.0%	100.0%	100.0%				
Total Brand				17,595	18,552	15,897	18,327	95	99	13.9	12.7
Share of Market				44.4%	48.7%	47.7%	53.5%				
Dinty Moore Beef Stew	7½ oz	24	0.41	3,790	3,773	1,475	1,555	46	47	6.2	6.1
Dinty Moore Beef Stew	15 oz	24	0.67	806	857	527	570	10	13	6.1	4.9
Dinty Moore Beef Stew	24 oz	24	0.96	9,145	8,566	8,467	8,239	83	87	8.5	7.5
Dinty Moore Beef Stew	40 oz	12	1.49	3,854	5,356	5,428	7,963	50	63	5.9	6.6
Total Brand				1,316	1,069	1,137	937	22	17	4.9	4.8
Share of Market				3.2%	2.4%	3.1%	2.3%				
Libby Beef Stew	16 oz	24	0.65	386	329	245	214	6	5	4.6	5.5
Libby Beef Stew	24 oz	12	0.98	930	740	892	723	18	17	4.0	3.2

TABLE 6 NEIS Data Services for Identifying Significant Consumer Buying Trends

1. Price (Lower/Higher)
2. Package (Convenience/Durability/Novelty)
3. Brand (National, Regional vs. Controlled)
4. Type (Moist/Dry—Chunky/Regular)
5. Size (Larger/Smaller)
6. Formula (With Borax/Ammonia—With Raisins/Dates)
7. Nutrition (Natural Ingredients/All Beef)
8. Convenience (Instant Breakfasts/Spray Cleaners)
9. Flavor/Color/Design (BBQ Flavor/Floral Print Design)
10. Diet (Low-Calorie/Cholesterol)
11. Ecology (Regular vs. Recyclable)

we mean private label, chain's own, or brands such as TOPCO, which, for example, may be marketed by two different chains—one in Cleveland and one in Kansas City—but are exclusive to these chains in their respective areas. These controlled brands are reported in the same detail as other brands—size, type, etc.—but not identified by chain—only as "controlled brands."

Other trends that are also identifiable through our Data Services report may relate to nutrition, convenience, diet, or be ecologically based on container type.

Although clients often purchase Data Services alone, many utilize it in conjunction with Nielsen Product Pickup Service, since by means of the pickup service it is possible to obtain samples of new products just introduced into the market.

As the name indicates, Product Pickup Service is just that; it's a facility for obtaining samples of any grocery product introduced into the market—at any place or at any time.

By means of 350 field agents, covering all principal cities and the areas between, we can supply one sample unit, or many hundreds of cases, of a specific brand to our clients. We are prepared to handle all perishable products—frozen, fresh, or other fragile items—and ship them anywhere, in special containers whenever necessary.

We can pick them up on a regular schedule—weekly, monthly, quarterly—or on a one-time-only basis. We can also secure samples in 23 additional countries through our overseas companies.

Over the years, we have obtained retail samples for an ever-widening variety of reasons or purposes. Table 7 lists a few of the more common reasons. They vary from wanting to check a competitive product for any number of reasons to qualitative assurance reasons relative to taste, flavor, color, freshness, nutrition maintenance, and so forth.

TABLE 7 Some Reasons for Using Nielsen Product Pickup Services

1. Competitive Products—New and Established
2. Average Age of Shelf Product
3. Taste and Flavor
4. Color
5. General Appearance—Label, Contents, etc.
6. Nutrition Maintenance

One of the more interesting programs we are now conducting is for the Food and Drug Administration, which utilizes the resources of not only Data Services and Product Pickup, but also our Food Index Service. The key here was Nielsen's unique ability to provide accurate market data coupled with a highly trained, nationwide field force capable of handling in-store assignments.

Here's how these services are being used to solve a problem facing the FDA. They wanted to assess the extent to which nutritional labeling had been accomplished, on a category-by-category basis, and then to measure the growth of the nutritionally labeled items versus competing items not so labeled.

The FDA contracted for the Data Services Directory, and matching computer tape, covering the progress of 430 edible grocery product classes in which they were concerned with nutritional labeling. These in turn were regrouped into very broad categories such as products containing flour, canned vegetables, dairy products, and so forth. Using the flour category as an example, they grouped all items in which flour was the primary ingredient—thus including pancake mixes, cake mixes, all-purpose flour, cookie mixes, etc. These broad categories were classified relative to contribution to total food sales, then each product class was ranked relative to its importance within the broad category. And finally, each individual brand was ranked relative to its importance within its product class.

Once these listings were completed, the FDA, by means of a sampling procedure, developed a brand listing of retail samples from each category to be secured from supermarkets. This listing was passed on to Nielsen's Product Pickup Service's central headquarters in Northbrook for fulfillment.

A number of leading brands on the list with virtually 100 percent distribution could be found in almost any supermarket and presented no problem. On the other hand, a good many others were regional or were fairly obscure brands with limited distribution.

To secure retail samples of these brands, we returned to the data bank and found the cities and areas where these brands were in distribution. From then on it was a simple matter to transmit pickup orders to the field agents in the respective areas and cities to secure the brand samples needed. Here is another example of the advantages of store-by-store data. In this case it was simply to retrieve shelf samples quickly and at low cost. But most often it is to determine what is happening, in what marketplace, and often why.

From these samples, the FDA is currently sorting out:

1. The brands requiring nutritional labels and, in fact, so labeled, from—
2. The brands requiring nutritional labels but not bearing them.
3. The brands *not* requiring nutritional labels but bearing them anyway.
4. Those *not* requiring nutritional labels and not having them.

Once all of the brands are placed in the proper groups, the FDA will go back to the Data Services Directory to establish the current dollar volume of each classification. To determine future growth, they will continue to monitor each group for the next year to assess gains and losses for each of the four.

In addition to the above, the FDA is also using the product samples to check whether the contents match the contents' label in terms of water, solids, etc. And, if the label carries a picture of the contents, does the picture truly represent the contents?

Another use of the product samples by the FDA is to run a nutrient assay of each of the products bearing nutritional labels to see if the nutritional values claimed by the label are in fact true.

A fourth use of the samples, and related to the one above, is an in-depth analysis of all of the products labeled as "dietetic." If the label claimed the product contained only four calories and no sugar, the contents were analyzed to verify the label claim.

As we understand it, the USDA is going to perform similar analyses on any products containing meat—sandwich spreads, chili, canned meat, etc.—since the FDA has no jurisdiction over meat products.

I'd like to make one final comment on this overall study. As you probably know, many food products are delivered directly to the store and never move through a wholesaler's or chain warehouse. For example, close to 90 percent of all soft drinks are delivered directly to the store; many dairy items—milk, butter, cheese, ice creams—are handled in the same way. Most crackers, cookies, some frozen foods, and other specialty items are also store–door delivered. In order to provide data on all of these items, we utilized Nielsen Food Index Services since they cover all items, regardless of source or type of distribution.

Since what is happening in the marketplace is such an important factor in the marketing of any product, we added another service, Store Observation Service, to assess the elements that so often influence the customer's decision to buy or not buy.

Availability or distribution is perhaps the most critical of all from everyone's point of view—manufacturer, retailer, and customer. Is the product there, on the shelf, where it can be purchased?

But also important are the selling prices, your product and your competitors'; the number of shelf facings (i.e., Is it easily visible?); shelf location—What shelf, what section, and where is the section in the store; and, Is the product being promoted or featured, and if so, how?

These are the questions most often asked, but many others of equal importance can be handled by this service.

To answer questions such as these, Nielsen employs a nationwide field staff specifically trained for this work. The staff, 80 in total, are located in 50 standard metropolitan statistical areas, in all areas of the country. The administration of the service is centralized in Northbrook, as are all Nielsen services.

In your invitation offering us the opportunity to present "our wares" before you this afternoon, you also requested that we address ourselves to certain questions, the first being, What gaps exist in the data base?

Nielsen Food Index, Nielsen Major Markets, and Nielsen Early Intelligence Service samples are all drawn from a universe with the following definition: all grocery stores, as defined by the U.S. Census Bureau, plus supermarket departments of general merchandise stores, i.e., the full-line grocery sections in mass merchandisers. This definition leaves out fringe-type stores handling small amounts of packaged groceries.

This measurement gap, expressed in terms of consumer grocery products, could be estimated for a typical product category to be 5 percent. Nielsen Early Intelligence System's Data Service's samples do not include small grocery stores. Since these small stores account for approximately 15 percent of total dollar volume, this could raise the gap for NEIS to close to 20 percent.

How complete are the data? I believe this can be answered in the following summary of Nielsen services:

- Nielsen Food Index Services—including Major Market Service—provide consumer sales plus retail inventories, purchases, distribution, out-of-stock, the prices paid by consumers, in-store promotional data, and retailer advertising.
- Data Services provide product movement to a sample of supermarkets. From this source, data are produced covering brand movement in both dollars and units per week per store, shares, distribution, and retail prices, and all brand details are broken down by size, flavor, type, and so forth.
- Product Pickup Service is a complete service and limited only by the client's desires. Store Observation Service, as the name implies, is based on observable data in the selling area of the store.

How reliable are the data? Samples for these services are drawn from a sampling frame defined in Table 1. Practically maximum geographical dispersion is achieved since, as an example, the 1,300-store national sample is spread through 606 counties. Similar dispersion is achieved in smaller areas sampled.

Quinquennial Census material, updated with material from the Census Bureau Current Retail Trade Programs, is used both to determine the sampling frame and to estimate universe data from sample results.

Sampling list material on a current basis is obtained from:

- progressive grocer lists,
- chain lists, and
- gathered by survey.

Sample units are selected with disproportionate sampling rates with larger stores having the greater chance of selection over small stores. This difference in selection rates is taken into consideration when sample data are projected to universe estimates.

At the same time that stores are audited to obtain data on individual grocery products, total retail dollar movement is obtained for each store for the audit period. This dollar movement is combined with the individual grocery product data to form a ratio. This ratio, having less variance from store to store than the absolute product data to be measured, gives the estimating process higher efficiency.

In summary, the sample design and estimation process has the following characteristics:

1. a stratified sample design using practically maximum geographic dispersion;
2. disproportionate sampling with greater chance of selection for large stores; and
3. ratio estimation to achieve greater precision.

Finally, I would like to comment on what I believe are the advantages that distinguish Nielsen marketing research services from any other.

First, in most instances, the data produced flow from the marketplace and result from consumer actions. As such, when we report consumer sales, it means the products in question have been purchased by consumers, not merely moved out of a warehouse. It's the same with prices—these are the prices paid by consumers. The distribution measurements are made in the store, as are the retail inventories and the data relating to sales influencing factors.

Second, nearly all the services are based on scientifically drawn samples. We believe that samples provide the greatest value in terms of dollars expended, accuracy achieved, and breadth of data.

And last, because of our access to the stores making up the samples, we can achieve a flexibility that's impossible to provide otherwise. I believe the study we are currently doing for the FDA is a good example of that.

APPENDIX

B Background Papers for Workshop on Evaluation of Methods for Obtaining Food Consumption Data

Dietary Methodology

CHARLOTTE M. YOUNG

It is of interest to find two branches of government suddenly showing interest in dietary methodology and willing to invest some money in solution to its problems. Literally millions of dollars have been spent on research in which dietary data have been related to various measures of nutritional status. Often the significance of the dietary methods used has been relatively unknown, and it has been difficult to figure out why the method used was chosen. Thirty some years ago I remember questioning the basis for choosing dietary methods used in certain studies and finally concluded it usually seemed to be expediency. These observations led me into some feeble efforts at looking at dietary methodology, which we did, with no special funds, as a side issue to another study. At that point I left an active interest in the field in pursuit of seeking answers to other practical questions in human nutrition.

STATE OF THE ART

For years I have tried to encourage nutritionists to make contributions to this field. The "take" has been very limited. Much of the basic work was done 20 to 40 years ago. Though for 20 years there has been a great need for dietary methodology for epidemiological studies dealing with the relationship between dietary intake of an individual and his biochemical or health status, we have not come very far. Many reviews of various depth and value concerning dietary survey methods have been written. I shall not attempt to compete with these; instead, I have prepared a list of many of the reviews including symposia on the subject which occurred in the 1950's and 1960's. The reader may refer to these for details.

Recently I have been impressed that the government has become very interested in dietary methodology. You will find the extensive review of Burk and Pao (1976) as they contemplated the 1975 Household Food Consumption Survey, the most recent in a series made about every 10 years by the U.S. Department of Agriculture. It is my understanding that several other sections of the government wished through this study to be able to obtain dietary information on both households and individuals. Hence in about 1975–76 the Consumer and Food Economics Institute of the USDA contracted with Response Analysis of Princeton, N.J., to do an extensive field trial after suggesting a series of methodologies to be tested. As I recall, the task was twofold: (1) to recommend procedures for a nationwide study of household food use and individual food intake with justification for such recommendations and (2) to recommend whether a pilot study was needed before proceeding with the nationwide data collection, together with a rationale for the conclusion reached. In this study some nine different methods received field trials. Eight of the methods included an effort to get information on household food usage by either some form of 7-day recall, diary, or interviews requiring different types of preparation or training. Four of the methods included data on individual family members using diary or recall for 1 to 3 days from the homemaker for all individuals in the household or from each individual subject as respondent. If the reports can be made available to you, the Committee and its consultants might well wish to examine them. None of the methods proposed incorporated a direct way of measuring its validity or reliability, since there was no observation of all food used or repeat observations in the same households. The Response Analysis survey is probably the most comprehensive study on dietary methodology of which I am aware. It is interesting that so quickly after these studies the Food and Drug Administration has asked the Food and Nutrition Board to conduct an in-depth study with some of the same directions. Such opportunities were what some of us dreamed of years ago. Today it is fortunate that diverse professions have developed interest in dietary methodology so that your Committee will have access not only to the talents of nutritionists of various backgrounds, but also epidemiologists, anthropologists, economists, sociologists, physicians, statisticians and computer scientists.

DIETARY STATUS, NOT NUTRITIONAL STATUS

It is imperative to remember that in measuring *dietary* status one is not measuring nutritional status. In using dietary assessments one should be quite clear as to their limitations, realizing that dietary studies give no *direct* measurement of nutritional status. They give only presumptive evidence. If food intake is quite poor, nutritional status *may* be below desirable limits. If nutrient intake appears to meet certain dietary standards and if the individual has no factors that may adversely condition his nutritional needs, he probably will be well nourished. Dietary studies should be referred to as diet studies, not nutritional studies.

In interpreting dietary information, one must bear in mind that there are pronounced individual differences in nutritional requirements; that our knowledge of absolute nutritional requirements is relatively meager; that a whole series of factors may condition an individual's nutrient needs by either interfering with the ingestion, absorption, or utilization of a nutrient or by increasing his nutritional needs through increased requirements, excretion, or destruction of the nutrient. These so-called "conditioning factors" may be discovered by medical histories and examination as part of a nutritional assessment but may be completely unknown in a dietary study. Furthermore, we have little information on how slight differences in nutrient intake affect the health of individuals, as well as little knowledge as to what level of failure to meet dietary allowances food intake affects the health of the individual. Additional laboratory and clinical tests are necessary before nutritional status is established.

Given these limitations, dietary studies do have many uses. In survey work alone, a description of food intake may be valuable in interpreting nutritional findings. The studies help to identify apparent dietary deficiencies or excesses. They also form a concrete basis for action programs, for in the long run, therapy will need to be interpreted into feeding programs. Also, valid and reliable information on dietary intake of an individual over a sufficient period of time may be important in relation to various biochemical and clinical measurements of his nutritional status.

AREAS IN WHICH WORK IS STILL NEEDED

Though there is need for work in the entire field of dietary methodology, certain areas stand out as especially critical:

1. *Validity*, which to my understanding does not include the refinements or subdivisions of Burk and Pao. To me, validity means the degree to which the method is a true measure of what the investigator wishes to describe. What one wishes to measure of course depends upon one's objectives. Burk and Pao describe five aspects of validity: accuracy, concurrent, construct, content, and predictive validities. The aspect most usually considered I suspect would come under *content* validity, i.e., does the method give the

"usual" picture of the subject's eating at the time in which the investigator is interested.

Too little information is available on validity, and probably "true" validity cannot be measured. In the early studies efforts were made to determine if two or more different methods gave comparable results or whether similar population samples in the same frame of time gave similar results. In more recent and sophisticated times, there have been an extremely limited number of studies in which *actual* intake (observed without the subject's knowledge) has been compared to the reported intake—whether by some form of record by the subject or by recall interview. Some have only been of a single meal. The ethical question always arises as to whether the subject should be aware that he is being observed. Factors that interfere with getting the desired "usual" picture include: (a) the tendency to eat differently during a record period either deliberately or unconsciously as a matter of convenience; (b) the desire to please or outwit the surveyor, which can lead either to omitting certain items or reporting certain foods the subject believes he should eat; (c) the general attitude to the questioner or to surveys in general; (d) ability or willingness to keep accurate records; (e) the condition of the subject's memory or willingness to use it; (f) food choice if the subject knows he is being observed; and (g) the mere act of record-keeping. Some individuals, such as homemakers, certain kinds of students, or certain food faddists, may be much more aware of what they eat than others.

2. *Reliability*, which to me means repeatability or true reproducibility or the error variation in collecting and processing dietary data. Some people confuse reliability as I am using it with validity. Most reliability studies have related to such matters as how accurately actual intake has been reported, errors due to the use of food tables, the differences in nutritional value between calculated and chemically analyzed diets, whether reported studies on the same population in a limited period of time gave similar results, and errors in sampling as induced by failure to get random samples when the objective would indicate its desirability but practical circumstances preclude random sampling.

3. *Intraindividual variability* in food or nutrient *intake*, which is especially important in determining the length of time that an individual needs to be studied for a true picture of intake be it current or past. There are more of these studies than those related to validity, but they still are quite limited.

4. *Interindividual variability,* which is of particular interest in population studies or group averages to determine the size of sample needed for the purpose. More has been done here than in the case of intraindividual variability.

In recent years the role of a statistician in the *planning* stages of a study as well as the later analytical stages has been appreciated by nutritionists.

Statisticians are extremely valuable in making the investigator clearly define his objectives and then in assisting in the many decisions that must be made such as sampling methods, sample size, appropriate quality control, setting up appropriate analyses, and interpretations of the results once available.

5. *Changes in inter- and intraindividual variability* over time and particularly in relation to seasonal variation.

6. *Epidemiological methods suitable for large-scale surveys* of the relationship of certain dietary or nutrient intakes or habits to disease conditions, two of which are of great current interest: coronary heart disease and cancer. Since such studies are often based on relatively large numbers of subjects, special techniques need to be developed or others adapted to the purpose. Five or six groups have attempted to develop various forms of short questionnaires and to check their validity and reliability. Hankin and her colleagues in a period of over 10 years (first in California and later in Hawaii) have developed and tested such a questionnaire in relation to cardiovascular disease, and more recently, to cancer. Previous techniques have been expensive and tedious and often could not be applied to all kinds of population groups. Also, often they have concentrated on only one facet of dietary pattern, i.e., the level of nutrient intake, with little information on other parameters of food intake such as specific food usage, changes in food patterns, spacing or apportionment of food over the day, environment, speed of eating, etc.

7. Need for more studies of *response rates* and factors that affect them.

8. Need for *studies of actual time and costs* involved in the use of different methods.

9. Development of methods for *use by relatively untrained, inexperienced interviewers,* or nonnutritionists.

10. The *role of different disciplines* in the study of dietary habits. The role of the statistician was mentioned earlier, but what about the others? We must recognize our need for them at appropriate times as well as their need in certain studies for the advice of an expert nutritionist. It is again part of the increasing recognition of the interdisciplinary nature of much research concerned with very personal aspects of human beings.

WHAT WE HAVE LEARNED; DECISIONS TO BE MADE

First and foremost, it is clear that the *objectives* of the dietary study must be clearly defined, for the objective determines the appropriate methods to be used in collecting, processing and interpreting the dietary data. Past studies would indicate that this point has not always been appreciated.

Secondly, it is clear on the basis of past dietary studies that there is a need for a clear-cut distinction between methods to be used for the *average intake of a group* for group comparisons and those suitable for defining the dietary intake of an *individual*. Dietary methodology studies have demonstrated the much smaller cost in time, money, and subject cooperation to obtain the mean intake of a group. There has been increasing realization of the time, cost, subject cooperation, and degree of precision necessary to obtain a valid and reliable measure of the intake of an individual.

Even after the objective is clearly defined, many decisions must be made with regard to methodology before a dietary study is undertaken, particularly studies concerned with the intake of individuals. Decisions with regard to the collection of data center on sampling, the schedule or form to be used and/or the interviewer, the instructions or supervision to be given, the time period to be covered, the timing of the recording process or recall period, the methods to be used in determining the amounts of food used, and whether food intake only or food habits as well are of interest.

Questions of sample size and type are fundamental. Does the sample need to be random so that one can describe a larger universe from which the sample was drawn? What limitations will be imposed by variation in the willingness of selected subjects to cooperate? Or can the sample be nonrandom if one is concerned with data on only the sample individuals and the characteristics of the larger universe bearing upon food consumption? The *size* of the sample varies with the objective and the method chosen but also on the classifications to be made in analyzing the data. For group averages a larger sample may be needed to include interindividual variability; the lower the variability in food consumption, the smaller the number needed for stable averages. The method of sampling should be clearly stated as well as information relative to those unwilling to or unable to cooperate. Too often this point has been neglected in reports. It is well to remember that sampling is a field of statistics in itself.

What time period should be covered? Are we interested in current intake, immediately past intake for a fixed period, or the usual or characteristic intake over an extended period in the present or past?

In what kind of dietary information are we interested? In nutrients, which ones? Foods? If so, which ones? Are we concerned with quantitative aspects or only the presence or absence of certain foods in the diet? Is it a food pattern in which we are interested? Are we concerned with food habits such as time, place, and circumstances of eating; with whom, regularity, food patterns, seasonings, waste, peculiarities of preparation, etc.?

How will amounts be reported? By weight, by household measures, by estimations of size of portions, or merely by the frequency with which some item is eaten? From whom shall such information be obtained, i.e., who will be the respondent? The individual subject, the person responsible for the subject's food, or both, or an observer? If the latter, what kind of training is needed?

The major determinant of these decisions is the objective of the study, but also to be considered are the resources available in terms of time, money, trained personnel, and the availability of a sufficient supply of suitable subjects (in Burk and Pao's terms, the respondent burden, field survey costs, and data-processing costs).

NECESSITY FOR PRETESTING METHODOLOGY

All evidence points to the necessity of pretesting the method on the particular population before undertaking a large study. As indicated earlier, possible methods vary with age, sex, culture, and education of the subjects as well as the complexity of the food resources available to the participant. Age is a factor not only for the very young, who cannot write or report, but also for the elderly, where memory may be affected. Education and culture may affect the ability to write and how much interviewers must be involved.

Inter- and intraindividual variability should be determined as an indication of the number of subjects needed as well as the time period that must be covered. It is also an opportunity to determine if there is a seasonal variation in intake. All too often the results are disastrous when pretesting has not been done. Quality control for data collection with training of interviewers and careful standardization must be planned.

In advance of the study, decisions also must be made with regard to methods of analysis, such as whether one is interested in diet patterns, frequency of intake of particular foods, or specific nutrients. If individual nutrients are to be calculated, what methods and what tables are suitable? If chemically analyzed, what methods? Interpretation or evaluation of adequacy then follows. For precision, even when food tables are used, there is increasing emphasis on chemical analyses of certain local foods to check values included in nationally used tables. Some investigators believe that before a major study is begun, the form of anticipated tables of results should be set up to be sure proper data and needed numbers of subjects are being used to meet the objective.

TYPES OF METHODS AVAILABLE

In general there are two types of dietary studies and within each type a variety of methods may be used: those concerned with food usage of families or institutions sharing common food supplies and those concerned with food usage of individuals. Information is obtained either by food records or by recall of what has been eaten.

Household or Institution Methods

Three methods are available:

1. *Food accounts*—a simple running description of food purchased, received as gifts, or produced for household use over a given period of time. These are not precise and rarely used today.
2. *Food records*—a weighted inventory of foods on hand at the beginning and close of the study together with a day-to-day record of food brought into the home or institution over the period of the study with or without an accounting of kitchen and plate waste or food fed to pets. This is the method the USDA used in its early household consumption studies.
3. *Food lists*—a method by which an interviewer obtains from the person responsible for the food an estimate of the quantities of food used over a given period of time. This is the method used by the USDA in the more recent household food consumption studies.

The methods vary widely in cost of collecting and processing the data and to some extent the uses to which the data may be put. It is well to remember *that there is no merit in using a more elaborate or expensive method than is necessary to obtain the data needed to meet the defined objective of the study.*

Individual Methods

Dietary data on individuals are collected either (1) to obtain average nutrient intake, food intake, or food habits of *groups* for comparison with other groups or (2) to obtain nutrient intake of a given *individual* for correlation with clinical or biochemical measurements obtained on that individual.

Studies vary from a qualitative type of food habit inquiry to those of a very much more precise quantitative nature. Each type of study has its use; the important thing is to consider carefully what kind of facts are needed for a given purpose and which method provides these facts at the lowest cost. Methods used with individuals include the following:

1. *An estimation* by recall, in which the subject, or in the case of young children perhaps the parent, recalls the food intake over the previous 24 hours or longer, with dependence on memory.
2. *Records* of food eaten by an individual kept by weights, household measurements, or by estimated quantities over a stated period of time.
3. *Dietary history*, in which by recall or repeated food records or both the interviewer aims to discover the usual eating patterns over a relatively long

period of time. It is a time-consuming process requiring professional personnel.

4. More recently *food frequency questionnaires,* either self-administered or interviewer-administered, have been studied as a means of acquiring information on general dietary intake or specific foods or nutrients over a longer period of time at less expense and with less personnel resources for epidemiological studies in which people may be grouped in extremes of intake. Unfortunately, a number of these initial efforts have not been done with typical American cultures.

5. *Weighted intake* for precise measurements during which all food eaten is carefully weighted and nutritive value either calculated from food tables or determined by laboratory analysis of duplicate samples; usually this method is used only in research groups with special facilities for collection and analysis.

FACTORS INVOLVED IN CHOICE OF METHODS OR STATE OF THE ART WITH REGARD TO EACH METHOD

Three statements of Keys (1968, 1979) may well be borne in mind as we consider the factors involved in choice of method. The first is that good surveys are difficult, costly, and require professional expertise in planning, operation, and interpretation. The second is that little is known of the long-time intraindividual variability of diet or that diet at any one time is representative over longer periods of time; and third, that even the best dietary surveys cannot provide answers about biochemical relationships.

Many comments may be made about the various dietary methods based on heterogenous dietary methodology studies that have been made over the last 40 years. More than most reviewers, Burk and Pao (1976) have brought them together in one place in relation to each type of method and is the latest review now in print. Hence the following discussion draws heavily on their review. Greater detail may be found in the review itself.

Food Accounts

This method is not widely used in this country. Great Britain and Israel are two countries with considerable experience with the method. In general, the food account gives a record of food entering the house or institution in a given period but not whether it is actually consumed in that period. It is less accurate than other household or institution methods but is felt by reviewers to give a good picture of the general diet. There is usually no indication of food discarded for spoilage, plate waste, other waste or fed to animals.

Sampling can be large since less is demanded of respondents. However, sampling is dependent on the willingness and the ability of the household to keep a written record (Sudman and Ferber, 1971). It is reported in one study that the lowest cooperation was found in one- or two-member households or where the head of the household was 55 years or older, or where there was less than an eighth grade education or income less than $2,000. Such households might be suspicious of surveys or find record-keeping difficult or too time-consuming. Though recording is not as detailed and time-consuming as other record methods, not all families will participate or are able to do so. It is possible that the diet is less likely to be altered by the food account method than by other more intrusive methods.

Little information is available on the respondent burden or field survey costs except that two or three visits per week are made to homes by field personnel. No data are available on processing costs.

Food Records

Information with regard to food record and list recall methods comes largely from studies done by the USDA, which has used the methods widely and has changed for its 10-year food consumption studies from the use of the food record (referred to by Burk and Pao as inventory record method) to the list recall method.

Inventory record and list recall procedures have been compared in unpublished studies by Murray (1970) and Grossman and Popka (1976). The latter provides the best basis for appraisal of the two methods. The reader is referred to the Burk and Pao review for details of the studies too extensive to be given here.

The food record method requires both considerable respondent cooperation and considerable interviewer time since food inventories must be taken previous to the onset of the record-keeping period and at the end of it. Records must be kept of all food entering the household during the specified period as well as quantities in weight and price expenditures.

Random sampling of households using this method is difficult or almost impossible, and therefore results cannot usually be generalized. The nonresponse rate is much higher than the list recall method, and fewer small and elderly households are likely to participate. Sampling is disturbed not only by the initial refusal to participate, but also by failure to keep the records once started and by incompleteness of the reporting of key items.

In one study it is reported that the quantity of food, money value, and nutritive values obtained with the food record method averaged 20 percent less than those derived from the list recall procedures. For these methods there is no direct comparison to actual values; comparison between methods is the best information available.

As to reliability, it is reported that based on quantities of major food groups food records and list recall give similar values. However, the list recall method gives slightly higher percentage standard errors. As to its repeatability it has been reported that similar mean values for food consumption have been obtained by replication of surveys.

As to validity, there is the problem of possible changes in food patterns because of the burden of weighing and measuring, or conforming to perceived culturally approved patterns.

Considerably higher field survey costs are involved with the food record due to the use of more interviewer time for the beginning and ending inventories and the visits in between, the total average time given as 5¾ hours.

There are also greater costs of processing data since some 12 hours were taken to prepare records for computer versus only about 5¼ hours for the recall schedules. Also it was reported that there were 3.7 times as many editing and processing errors per set of food records as per list recall schedules.

Some reviewers make the point that in Europe weighing of ingredients rather than use of household measurements is fairly common, and consequently there may be fewer problems with the food record method. In any case, the lower respondent rate in sampling is a major handicap in the use of the family or institution food record method.

Food List or List Recall

The food list or list recall method usually involves only one visit by the interviewer and is reported to take an average of 2 hours if no memory aids are involved or 2½ hours if memory aids are used. A major advantage is a higher response rate so that a more adequate and representative sample may be attained than in the case of the food record method. Small households and older households are reported as more likely to respond to the list recall method.

Burk and Pao indicate that researchers experienced in surveying homemakers for food data insist most homemakers are able to recall household use between two time boundaries if they are related to the cycle of food activities. Furthermore, major food shopping has been shown to be done by the week, or less often, and usually by the homemaker. The method also has the advantage that the interviewer can immediately evaluate responses and probe for additional information when needed. Quality and completeness of information such as sizes of containers, brands, etc., can be improved by the interchange between interviewer and respondent and observation at the home site.

It is interesting that the use of memory aids seemed to annoy many respondents, and, in a comparison of list recall interviews where memory aids were used in contrast to where they were not, little effect was shown on the amounts recalled.

As indicated earlier, the field survey costs were lower for the list recall method since the average interviewer time was less than half that for the food record method. One would wonder, too, if costs would not be less in achieving the desired respondent rate because of the lower response rate for the food record method.

The computer-related processing costs were less than half for the list recall method as for the food record method; in addition, much more time was spent to rectify the greater number of editing and processing errors per set of food record schedules as contrasted to the list recall schedule.

Thus, in this country for household or institutional studies the list recall method in recent years has taken precedence over the food record method, particularly in government circles (USDA, 1972b).

INDIVIDUAL METHODS

Burk and Pao conclude that no one method is consistently advantageous over all others and that researchers have to decide what trade-offs are most relevant to their objectives.

Recall

The 24-hour recall is often used to get a general diet pattern on a group basis; it has the disadvantage of relying on memory. However, memory for recalls limited to 24 hours appears quite good except perhaps in older people. Campbell and Dodds (1967) found there was a significant difference between older and younger subjects in calories forgotten and that the factor of age was more important than education. They concluded that before the shorter, more economical 24-hour recall is used with older people where the menu is not known, modifications will be needed if reliable data are to be obtained. They suggest that a checklist or the assistance of a spouse or younger family member may be required.

The 24-hour recall is particularly good for group studies because it saves the risk of individuals changing their customary food patterns and, in most cases, because of the higher response rate due to the light respondent burden. There is the problem of the subject's inability to estimate certain sizes accurately, which may be helped to some extent by the interviewer's use of models, glasses, bowls, and spoons of various sizes to aid in the estimation of portion sizes. There are problems of both under- and overestimation and some report a greater tendency toward underestimation of intakes.

A great advantage is the greater response rate, which, on a group basis, gives greater representative and predictive validity. Also costs are lower because of less personnel time, though processing costs will be higher to convert estimates to weights.

On an individual basis, the place of the 24-hour recall still needs to be established. Obviously, the 24-hour recall of intake cannot be correlated with clinical or biochemical measurements on the individual that result from intake over a much longer period of time. It is conceivable that repeated 24-hour recalls over a substantial period of time might be useful for this purpose.

Reliability as related to sampling appears to be high in terms of satisfactory samples obtained (Abraham *et al.*, 1974; Swanson *et al.*, 1959; USDA, 1972a) though less satisfactory samples have been reported by others (Morgan, 1959; USDHEW, 1972).

Reliability (repeatability) has been good in terms of actual consumption for groups of children (Emmons and Hayes, 1973; Samuelson, 1970) with advance notice helping recall (Meredith *et al.*, 1951). The same study indicated more underreporting with increased number of items with 86 hospitalized lactating women. Linusson *et al.* (1974), comparing recall information with quantities eaten at all three meals as determined by weighing by the interviewer, found the recall method appeared fairly accurate for qualitative estimation of averages for population groups but not highly valid for ascertaining quantity of food consumed. Regression analyses between recall and actual intake showed for all food groups a tendency to overestimate actual intake when consumption was low and to underestimate it when it was high.

In a study by Gersovitz *et al.* (1978), the internal validity of a 24-hour recall and 7-day dietary record was investigated among a group of noninstitutionalized *elderly* subjects who were participating in a congregate meals plan. Internal validity was assessed by comparing reported intake with unobtrusively obtained data on actual intake for the single meal per day at the congregate meal site. Paired test results for both the 24-hour recall and the 7-day record suggest that both methods provide equally accurate estimates of the mean intake. Results suggested that the recall is prone to *over*reporting *low* intakes and *under*reporting *high* intakes, a pattern referred to as the "flat slope syndrome," the main implications of which are a downward bias in the number of subjects with extremely high or extremely low intakes.

Balogh *et al.* (1971) in Israel with volunteer male clerical and administrative workers found that repeated 24-hour recalls were valuable aids in the difficult and complex area of classifying individual dietary intakes and should be used more frequently, particularly for those populations and for those specific nutrients for which the range of variability is not extreme. They state that when variability *is* extreme, the method of repeated 24-hour recall interview will reveal the situation and point toward the hard fact that no method short of extensive daily sampling is likely to be successful in accurately categorizing large numbers of individuals with respect to dietary intake.

Frank *et al.* (1977) have proposed an improved 24-hour recall technique to be used with school children that requires well-trained nutritionists, graduated food models, and standardized probing. Two different nutritionists as interviewers for the same children produce results that are not significantly different. The interview, however, took 30 to 40 minutes per child.

Madden *et al.* (1976), using a sample of subjects 60 years or older, compared actual intake with 24-hour recall intakes. By paired test no significant difference was found between mean recall and mean actual intake for any of eight nutrients except calories. Using regression analysis, results indicated that for calories, protein, and vitamin A small intakes tended to be overreported and large intakes underreported.

According to Burk and Pao's classification, the accuracy aspect of validity, i.e., the absence of systemic error, found that for group averages the 24-hour recall could substitute for an estimated 7-day record (Young *et al.*, 1952b). Adelson (1960) found the 7-day record of intelligent adult men gave similar results to the 7-day weighed records. However, Trulson (1954) found recalls by children gave lower averages than 7-day estimated records. Campbell and Dodds (1967) found evidence of underestimation but the ability to remember in their older subjects increased by probing.

Burk and Pao's concurrent validity, i.e., two measures of the same concept, examines studies of weighed records in relationship to recalls. Bransby *et al.* (1948) with school boys in Britain, and Thomson (1958) with pregnant women in Britain, found recalls gave lower estimates and, for Bransby *et al.*, in some cases higher. Adelson (1960) for adults, and Samuelson (1970) for children in Sweden, found acceptable comparisons between the two.

In construct validity, i.e., the degree to which variability in concept is measured, for various groups of children (Eppright *et al.*, 1952); Iowa, South Dakota, and North Central women (Swanson *et al.*, 1959); USDA unpublished data (1965); and HANES data on women age 60 and over (Abraham *et al.*, 1974), relative standard errors depended somewhat on group size, but 24-hour recall compared favorably with estimated record.

For representative validity, i.e., the measure or level taken as an indicator of a more general level, the 24-hour recall appeared to yield better representation than other methods, because response rates were higher (Mongeau, 1974).

For predictive validity, the good response rate for 24-hour recall contributes to its usefulness (USDA, 1972a).

Response burden is lightened by the use of the 24-hour recall (Young *et al.*, 1952b) and field survey costs are less if only one visit is necessary (Adelson, 1960); data-processing costs are increased when household measures must be converted to weights (Adelson, 1960).

Records (Estimated)

Response rate for the dietary record method is apt to be less than the 24-hour recall, because some people will not take on the burden of record-keeping and some may be unable to keep records.

Food survey costs will vary with the number of interviewer visits required. Data-processing costs include the necessity of converting estimated amounts to weights or to common household measures.

Some investigators believe that a 1-day record—in other cases, a 3-day record—will give a reliable average dietary intake of a group if enough individuals are included. However, they are not adequate for measurements for individuals. There is no common agreement on the period required in this case, and it does vary with which nutrients one wishes to measure. A 7-day record has been most commonly used, but there is evidence because of intraindividual variability and seasonal variability that it probably is not adequate. Longer periods are difficult to obtain and further reduce response rates. Very few long-term studies have been done (Chappell, 1955; Young *et al.*, 1953b; Yudkin, 1951).

For some population groups, the day of record-keeping as well as the day of the week makes a substantial difference. More research is needed on the number, spacing, and section of days of record-keeping. When greater variety of foodstuffs and smaller samples are used, longer periods of time are necessary. With limited variety of foods, shorter periods may be used.

The accuracy of estimated records may be questioned. One of the big handicaps in many estimated records is the inability of subjects to estimate portion sizes of food accurately particularly for certain types of food (Young *et al.*, 1953a).

Reliability as related to sampling is more difficult than for the 24-hour recall. A random sample is difficult to obtain because of the relatively low response rate though it is considered less difficult than the weighed record (Marr, 1971).

On a group basis, 1 day was considered satsifactory by Chalmers *et al.* (1952) with a variety of population groups, but others considered consecutive days to be necessary (Eppright *et al.*, 1955, 1972). Estimated records gave higher nutritive values than weighed records (Eppright *et al.*,

1952) but results by other investigators were inconsistent (Bransby *et al.*, 1948; Young *et al.*, 1953a). Still other investigators found correlation between consecutive days (Trulson, 1951), but Chalmers *et al.* (1952) found no correlation. Evidence of actual variability was found by Celender (1963) and Young *et al.* (1953b).

As far as accuracy is concerned there was an upward bias at the start as reported by Celender (1963) and Young *et al.* (1953a). Several studies report bias because of inability to estimate portion sizes accurately (Young *et al.*, 1953a); others indicate that some respondents are unwilling to report accurately (Paul *et al.*, 1963). Still others found accuracy was influenced by interviewers (Church *et al.*, 1954; Steele *et al.*, 1951). An effect of day of record-keeping was reported by Cellier and Hankin (1963), Eppright *et al.* (1952), and Leverton and Marsh (1939).

Eppright *et al.* (1952) and Owen *et al.* (1974) reported concurrent validity with positive correlation of dietary findings with biochemical measures.

In terms of construct validity Young *et al.* (1952b) found that for group averages a 1-day record was sufficient, but for the estimate of an individual's intake, a longer period is necessary. The length of time required varied with the particular nutrient.

In terms of representative validity, several investigators reported that consecutive 3-day records did not give the same results as 1 day, 7 days, or combinations of nonconsecutive days (Eppright *et al.*, 1952; Hankin *et al.*, 1967; Trulson, 1951). Others have shown that weekend days give different results than week days (Cellier and Hankin, 1963; Leverton and Marsh, 1939). Representativeness of data is also affected by the nonresponse rate of the sample as shown by Owen *et al.* (1974) in the national preschool nutrition survey.

Eppright *et al.* (1972), Owen *et al.* (1974), and other surveys have demonstrated good predictive validity of food and nutrition intake measured with estimated records.

Response rate is reduced when the estimated food record method is used because of the burden to the subject as demonstrated by both Mongeau (1974) and Young *et al.* (1952b).

Field survey costs are increased if more than one interviewer visit is required (Eppright *et al.*, 1972; Owen *et al.*, 1974), and data-processing costs are increased when household measures must be converted to weights or common measures.

Dietary History

The dietary history method was developed by Burke (1947) as a research tool to estimate usual or average food and nutrient intake over a period of time so it might be related to growth or other clinical measurements. The rationale was that such measurements are the result of earlier, long-time food habits, not current habits alone. As used by Burke and later her student, Beal (1967), in growth and development studies of children, repeated dietary studies were done on the same children and were useful in classifying them into groups. Both 3-day records and recall of usual intake starting with the past 24 hours were used together with subsequent cross-check with a food list partially as a means of probing. Their subjects usually knew in advance histories were to be taken and therefore were alerted to being more aware of their food intake than has been the case of some subsequent uses of the method. Having observed Burke taking dietary histories with her quiet, nonsuggestive method, which put the subject at ease, I am convinced that in her hands it was quite different than has been practiced by others.

The method requires a highly skilled and trained interviewer and usually takes an hour or longer to obtain. Obviously it cannot be done by just anyone with just any subject. In some cases of people with fairly unstructured eating patterns, it may be impossible. However, for long-term studies, or one concerned with immediate past intake, it is one of the few possibilities if skilled personnel and sufficient time are available.

Several investigators have been able to get satisfactory samples with the use of the dietary history method (Burke, 1947; Beal, 1967; Christakis *et al.*, 1968; Dawber *et al.*, 1962; Mann *et al.*, 1962; Young *et al.*, 1952a).

Results relative to repeatability have varied with different investigators and different types of subjects. Reshef and Epstein (1972) found good correlations for repeat interviews using the same nutritionist; Huenemann and Turner (1942) found that subjects really did not know what they ate. Good repeatability for group averages did not necessarily imply good estimates for individuals (Celender, 1963; Reed and Burke, 1954; Trulson and McCann, 1959). Several studies have shown that the diet history is likely to give higher estimates of intake than other methods (Young *et al.*, 1952b; Trulson, 1951; Stevens *et al.*, 1963; Celender, 1963). In some cases the subjects had not been alerted to being aware of their dietary intake.

Since in most cases the dietary history method has not been used with probability samples, it would rate poorly in terms of representativeness.

The respondent burden is little for the dietary history method but the effort is great for the interviewer (den Hartog *et al.*, 1965). Field survey costs are high in terms of needing highly skilled and specially trained nutritionists with approximately an hour or longer for each interview, and considerably longer to edit interviews and prepare them for data processing.

FOOD FREQUENCY METHOD FOR RECALL OR PAST FOOD INTAKE

Increasingly various forms of dietary questionnaires have been developed for use in epidemiologic studies to give an indication how often certain foods are eaten in a given period of time. These questionnaires may be given by interview or they may be self-administered. One of the earliest was developed by Stefanik and Trulson (1962), which took 20–25 minutes by interview. Results were compared with either recent 7-day records or previous dietary histories. The investigators felt at the group level and at the individual level of analysis the short questionnaire gave generally equivalent estimates of the qualitative consumption of foods.

Very shortly afterwards, Abramson *et al.* (1963) reported a study designed to determine if the frequency with which specific foods were taken might be a reasonable index of the usual quantity of these foods eaten per week; both sets of data were obtained by interview. They then tried to test the value of the method empirically by seeking associations between the frequency data and the subject's hemoglobin level. It was not possible to obtain quantitative data by actual measurement for comparison with the frequency data, and the reliability of the method, that is, the extent to which a repeated interview promoted similar information to the first, was not tested. Data were obtained from 30-minute interviews with a heterogeneous sample of 60 Jewish women aged 17 to 39 in the fifth and eighth months of pregnancy. The findings suggest that variations in size of average servings do not outweigh effects of differences in frequency. The authors felt that with the heterogeneous populations the food frequency interview did not give results close enough to quantitative intake to justify the choice of the method in studies of the diet of individuals, but it was close enough to warrant its consideration of moderately sizable groups in an epidemiologic study. A main limitation of the method they felt to be its inability to produce data on individual nutrients.

Balogh *et al.* (1968), in a long-term prospective investigation of ischemic heart disease of adult Israeli males 40 years and older, developed a short dietary questionnaire of 15 minutes duration. It was based on a scoring system of frequency × nutrients × amount and a week period. Estimation of portion size was aided by food models and a food list was used instead of meal patterns. The validity was tested with 49 persons against a modified Burke dietary history and a combined week's record with weighing of representative food items. The authors felt the questionnaire to be a practical tool for the assessment of dietary intake in the prospective study.

Epstein *et al.* (1970), in another Israeli study using groups of men and women, some born in North Africa and others in Europe, compared a short dietary questionnaire with a research dietary history of the Burke type. There was a moderate or low correlation between the data obtained by the same individuals by the two methods. The finding suggested that the validity of the short questionnaire method varied with sex, age, ethnic group, and education and was lowest among persons with a varied diet. The mean daily intake of nutrients was lower by the short method. The lack of high correlation between data obtained by the two methods was taken as evidence that the short questionnaire is not a very valid indicator of the diet of an individual. In 1972, Reshef and Epstein reported that the reliability of the questionnaire did not vary in the different sex and country of birth groups. None of the mean values for the food items was significantly different in two interviews. In addition, variability of the diet did not affect the reliability.

Browe *et al.* (1966a) reported the use of a questionnaire to estimate the dietary intake of 1,514 male civil service employees being followed in an epidemiologic study of cardiovascular disease in New York State. The survey was done to classify the men's diets in relation to serum lipid levels, other clinical data being gathered and subsequent occurrence and clinical course of heart disease. The advantages of the method include ease of administration, relatively low cost, minimum need for specially trained personnel, and ease of application to large-scale surveys. The disadvantages are mainly those typified by all nonobjective methods for assessing dietary intake.

Yudkin (1966) used a 15–20-minute clinic interview questionnaire with 23 heart patients to assess sugar intake. Comparison was made to 7-day food records in household measures made by the subjects a few days later. Yudkin felt the short questionnaire gave average results that agreed well with the 7-day records. Stead (1968) compared two different modifications of the Burke dietary history method for estimate of average nutrient intake of a group of 30 white 12-year-old school girls in Pretoria. The results obtained by the two methods agreed fairly well in the case of almost all nutrients studied.

Hankin and others have worked with developing a self-administered short questionnaire to estimate accurately the dietary intakes of participants in cardiovascular epidemiologic studies in San Francisco with Japanese-American men and later in Honolulu since 1967 (Hankin and Huenemann, 1967; Hankin *et al.*, 1967; Hankin *et al.*, 1970) and later for studies of gastrointestinal cancer (Hankin *et al.*, 1975; Hankin *et al.*, 1978). The questionnaires were based on 7-day measured food records. In formulating the questionnaires, food groups were used. For group purposes a limited number of food items that took 30 minutes per questionnaire predicted fairly well the average intake of the men for the nutrients considered. To use the method, a preliminary investigation with a sample of the population to be studied is necessary to establish standards, to identify particular items eaten in definable serving units, and to provide data for comparable regression equations appropriate to the population.

WEIGHED RECORD METHOD

A weighed record is a history of all foods eaten by an individual in a specified period with the amounts of each determined by weighing. It is a most reliable and most expensive method and the only method for absolute accuracy of quantity of food eaten. But the weighing procedure limits the size of sample and tends to disrupt customary routines. It is most ideal for clinical studies; yet it can be used only for current intake and does not give information on long-term intakes. Since foods are in weighed portions, processing costs are less, but more personnel time may be involved in field survey costs.

No satisfactory evaluations of this method for large surveys were found in the literature using weighed and analyzed records, probably because of the great cost in time and money, need for literate and highly cooperative subjects and the small number of persons who can be handled (Marr, 1971; Mongeau, 1974). Random samples are very difficult to obtain because of low response rate (Burrill *et al.*, 1959; den Hartog *et al.*, 1965; Leverton and Pazur, 1957).

Greatest variation was found in day to day records, but 7 days was considered sufficiently reliable for group averages (Adelson, 1960; Widdowson, 1947). However, 1 week was not considered a reliable estimate of an individual's intake (Chappell, 1955; Fry *et al.*, 1963; Huenemann and Turner, 1942; Young *et al.*, 1952a, 1953; Yudkin, 1951).

From an accuracy aspect of validity, Marr (1971) considers the weighed record the most accurate measure. Yudkin (1951) felt there was an upward bias at the start, whereas den Hartog *et al.* (1965) and Ohlson *et al.* (1950) felt there was a downward bias if it was too much trouble for the respondent. If a portion size is missing an average size is inserted. Dieckmann *et al.* (1951), in a study of pregnant women, found weighed portion sizes did not conform to those postulated in printed tables, whereas Beegle *et al.* (1954) with a group of mature women found mean and median amounts eaten of any given food were relatively close. Use of food composition tables for nutrient content was found to give acceptable accuracy (Widdowson and McCance, 1943); others report less than acceptable accuracy (Leverton, 1937; Manalo and Jones, 1966; Walberg and Adams, 1965).

As far as concurrent validity is concerned, Eppright *et al.* (1952) found that averages for estimated records exceeded means from weighed records. However, Dieckmann *et al.* (1952) and Huenemann and Turner (1942) found positive correlations with biochemical measures.

As far as concurrent validity (i.e., the degree to which variability in concept is measured) is concerned, Marr (1971) stated that the weighed record gives a precise measure of intake, but not necessarily of customary consumption. In Italy (Fidanza and Fidanza-Alberti, 1967) and in England (Heady, 1961), researchers felt that records for 3–5 days capture most of the information. Keys *et al.* (1966) and Yudkin (1951) felt that less than 1 week was too short a period.

Representative validity because of the low response rates adversely affects generalization of results when the weighed record is used (Adelson, 1961; Thomson, 1958), and predictability is low for large-scale surveys.

The respondent burden for the weighed method is heavy (Eppright *et al.*, 1952; den Hartog *et al.*, 1965). Field survey costs are higher if more than one interviewer visit is required (Adelson, 1960; den Hartog *et al.*, 1965; Marr, 1971). However, data-processing costs are decreased because foods do not require conversion to common weights.

SUMMARY

There is obviously a need for more methodology studies, since there are still many unanswered questions. It is apparent from the diversity of results that pretesting is basic with the population group to be studied before a major survey is undertaken. It would be helpful if the results of such pretesting were made available in the literature. The greatest need is a means of finding out past individual intake for correlation with physical and biochemical measurements on the individual.

REFERENCES AND BIBLIOGRAPHY

Abraham, S., F. Lowenstein, and C. Johnson. 1974. Preliminary findings of the first health and nutrition examination survey, United States, 1971–72: Dietary intake and biochemical findings. U.S. Department of Health, Education, and Welfare, National Center for Health Statistics, Public Health Service. DHEW Publ. No. (HRA) 74-1219-1. 183 pp.

Abramson, J. H., C. Slome, and C. Kosovsky. 1963. Food frequency interview as an epidemiological tool. Am. J. Public Health 53:1093.

Adelson, S. F. 1960. Some problems in collecting dietary data from individuals. J. Am. Diet. Assoc. 36:453.

Adelson, S. F. 1961. Practical procedures for dietary surveys. Pages 85–96 *in* Proc. 3rd Intl. Congr. Dietet. Newman Books, London.

Adelson, S. F., E. Asp, and I. Noble. 1961. Household records of food used and discarded. A pilot study in St. Paul. J. Am. Diet. Assoc. 39:578.

Anderson, R. K., and H. R. Sandstead. 1947. Nutritional appraisal and demonstration program of the U.S. Public Health Service. J. Am. Diet. Assoc. 23:1201.

Assessment of nutritional status and food consumption surveys. 1974. *In* J. E. Somogyi, Ruschhkon-Zurich, and A. Szczygiel, eds. Proc. Eleventh Symp. Group Europ. Nutr. Warsaw, Apr. 9–13, 1972. Bibl. Nutr. Diet. 20.

Baker, H., O. Frank, S. Feingold, *et al.* 1967. Vitamins, total cholesterol and triglycerides in 642 New York City school children. Am. J. Clin. Nutr. 20:850.

Balogh, M., J. H. Medalie, H. Smith, and J. J. Groen. 1968. The development of a dietary questionnaire for ischemic heart disease survey. Isr. J. Med. Sci. 4:195.

Balogh, M., H. A. Kahn, and J. H. Medalie. 1971. Random repeat 24-hour dietary recalls. Am. J. Clin. Nutr. 24:304.

Bavly, S. 1976. Levels of nutrition in Israel, 1968–69. Family Expenditure Survey Part II. Ministry Educ. Culture, Coll. Nutr. Home Econ., Cent. Bur. Stat., Jerusalem. 102 pp.

Beal, V. A. 1967. The nutritional history in longitudinal research. J. Am. Diet. Assoc. 51:426.

Becker, B. G., B. P. Indik, and A. M. Beeualkes. 1960. Dietary intake methodologies—A review. Univ. Mich. Res. Inst. Tech. Rep. Proj. 03188, Ann Arbor, Mich.

Bebb, H. T., T. B. Houser, J. C. Witchi, and A. S. Littell. 1972. Nutritive content of the usual diets of 82 men. J. Am. Diet. Assoc. 61:507.

Beegle, R. M., P. H. Roberts, N. Howard, *et al.* 1954. Weights of foods eaten per meal by 242 women 30–92 years of age. Mich. Agric. Exp. Stn. Tech. Bull. 244, No.-Cent. Region. Publ. 37. 32 pp.

Bigwood, E. J. 1939. Guiding principles for studies on the nutrition of populations. League of Nations Health Organization, Geneva.

Bransby, E. R., C. G. Daubney, and J. King. 1948. Comparison of results obtained by different methods of individual dietary survey. Brit. J. Nutr. 2:89–110.

Browe, J. H., R. M. Gofstein, D. M. Morlley, and M. C. McCarthy. 1966a. Diet and heart disease study in the cardiovascular health center. 1. A questionnaire and its application in assessing dietary intake. J. Am. Diet. Assoc. 48:95.

Browe, J. H., D. M. Morlley, *et al.* 1966b. Diet and heart disease study in the cardiovascular health center, 2. Construction of a food table and its use. J. Am. Diet. Assoc. 48:101.

Browe, J. H., D. M. Morlley, V. M. Logrillo, and J. T. Doyle. 1967. Diet and heart disease study in the cardiovascular health center. 3. Dietary intake and physical activity of male civil service employees. J. Am. Diet. Assoc. 50:376.

Bryan, A. H., and E. L. Anderson. 1960. Retrospective dietary interviewing. A technique. J. Am. Diet. Assoc. 37:558.

Bureau of Human Nutrition and Home Economics. 1948. Summary of Proceedings of a Conference on the Study of Food Intake. U.S. Department of Agriculture, Washington, D.C., October 25–28, 1948. Mimeo.

Burk, M. C., and E. M. Pao. 1976. Methods for large scale surveys of household and individual diets. Home Econ. Res. Rep. No. 40. U.S. Government Printing Office, Washington, D.C., November 1976.

Burke, B. S. 1947. The dietary history as a research tool. Am. Diet. Assoc. J. 23:1041–1046.

Burrill, L. M., B. Alsup, C. Schuck, *et al.* 1959. Evaluation of the self-chosen weighted diets of 402 women 30–97 years of age in the seven North Central states. S. Dak. State Coll., Home Econ. Dept., Agric. Exp. Stn. Bull. 478, No.-Cent. Region. Publ. 105. 19 pp.

Campbell, V. A., and M. L. Dodds. 1967. Collecting dietary information from groups of older people. Am. Diet. Assoc. J. 51(1):29–33.

Celendar, I. H. 1963. Reliability of methods of recording dietary intake in women at constant weight. University Microfilms, Ann Arbor, Mich. 161 pp.

Cellier, K. M., and M. E. Hankin. 1963. Studies of nutrition in pregnancy. I. Some considerations in collecting dietary information. Am. J. Clin. Nutr. 13:55–62.

Chalmers, F. W., M. M. Clayton, L. O. Gates, *et al.* 1952. The dietary record—How many and which days?

Chamberlain, K., and M. Pike. 1948. An experimental study of the accuracy of a method of survey of individual diets not directly based on weighing. Scientific Advisors Division, Ministry of Food, London. Mimeo to Author.

Chappell, G. M. 1955. Long-term individual dietary surveys. Br. J. Nutr. 9:323–339.

Christakis, G., A. Miridjanian, L. Nath, *et al.* 1968. A nutritional epidemiologic investigation of 642 New York City children. Am. J. Clin. Nutr. 21:107.

Church, H. N., M. M. Clayton, C. M. Young, and W. D. Foster. 1954. Can different interviewers obtain comparable dietary survey data? J. Am. Diet. Assoc. 30:777.

Clark, F. 1969. The 1965–66 food consumption survey: Scope, methodology, and highlights. Pages 43–56 *in* Using food surveys in consumer education. N.C. State Univ. Agric. Policy Inst., Raleigh.

Clark, F. 1974. Recent food consumption surveys and their uses. Fed. Proc. 33:2270.

Committee on Nutrition Surveys. 1949. Nutrition surveys: Their techniques and value. National Research Council, Bull. 117, National Academy of Sciences, Washington, D.C., May 1949. (See Section II, Dietary surveys and their interpretations, pp. 11–47.)

Darby, W. J. 1947. The influence of some recent studies in the interpretation of the findings of dietary surveys. J. Am. Diet. Assoc. 23:204.

Dawber, T., G. Pearson, P. Anderson, *et al.* 1962. Dietary assessment in the epidemiologic study of coronary heart disease: The Framingham study. II. Reliability of measurement. Am. J. Clin. Nutr. 11:226.

den Hartog, C., Th. Van Schaik, L. Dalderup, *et al.* 1965. The diet of volunteers participating in a long term epidemiological field survey on coronary heart disease at Zutphen, The Netherlands. Voeding 26:184.

Dieckmann, W. J., D. F. Turner, E. J. Meiller, *et al.* 1951. Observations on protein intake and health of mother and baby. II. Food intake. J. Am. Diet. Assoc. 27:1053.

Dierks, E. C., and L. M. Morse. 1965. Food habits and food intakes of preschool children. J. Am. Diet. Assoc. 47:292.

Dietary methodologies. 1973. *In* Nutritional assessment in health programs. Am. J. Public Health 63(Suppl.):11–18.

Durnin, J. V. G. A., and E. C. Blake. 1962. A comparison of the food intake of elderly women estimated by individual inventory and the National Food Survey methods. Br. J. Nutr. 16:261.

Eads, M. G., and A. P. Meredith. 1948. Nutrition studies. II. Methods of collecting dietary data. Public Health Rep. 63:777.

Eagles, J. A., M. G. Whiting, and R. E. Olson. 1966. Dietary appraisal. Problems in processing dietary data. Am. J. Clin. Nutr. 19:1.

Emmons, L., and M. Hayes. 1973. Accuracy of 24-hour recalls of young children. J. Am. Diet. Assoc. 62:409.

Eppright, E. S., M. B. Patton, A. Marlatt, and M. Hathaway. 1952. Dietary study methods. V. Some problems in collecting dietary information about groups of children. J. Am. Diet. Assoc. 28:43.

Eppright, E. S., E. Jebe, V. Sidwell, *et al.* 1955. Nutrition of 9-, 10- and 11-year-old public school children in Iowa, Kansas and Ohio. Iowa State Coll. Iowa Agric. Exp. Stn. Bull. 434:616.

Eppright, E. S., H. M. Fox, B. A. Fryer, *et al.* 1972. Nutrition of infants and preschool children in the north central region of the United States of America. World Rev. Nutr. Diet. 14:269.

Epstein, L. M., A. Reshef, B. Abramson, and O. Bialik. 1970. Validity of a short dietary questionnaire. Isr. J. Med. Sci. 6:589.

Exton-Smith, A. N., and R. R. Stanton. 1965. Report of an investigation into the diet of elderly women living alone. Edwards Hospital Fund for London.

Fidanza, F. 1971. Sources of error in dietary surveys. Bibl. Nutr. Dieta 1972. 20:105.

Fidanza, F., and A. Fidanza-Alberti. 1967. Dietary surveys in connection with the epidemiology of heart disease. Reliability, sources of variation, and other data from nine surveys in Italy. Voeding 28:244.

Flores, M. 1972. Methodology in nutrition surveys among preschool children. Arch. Latinoam. Nutr. 22:359.

Frank, G. C., G. S. Berenson, P. E. Schilling, and M. C. Moore. 1977. Adapting the 24-hr. recall for epidemiologic studies of school children. J. Am. Diet. Assoc. 71:26.

Fry, P. C., H. M. Fox, and H. Linkswiler. 1963. Nutrient intakes of healthy older women. J. Am. Diet. Assoc. 42:218.

Futrell, M. F., L. Kilgore, and F. Windham. 1971. Nutritional status of negro preschool children in Mississippi. Evaluation of HOP index. J. Am. Diet. Assoc. 59:218.

George, P. S., and G. A. King. 1961. Consumer demand for food commodities in the United States with projections for 1980. Calif. Univ. Agric. Sci., Giannini Found. Monogr. 26. 161 pp.

Gersovitz, M., J. P. Madden, and H. S. Wright. 1978. Validity of the 24-hr. dietary recall and seven-day record for group comparisons. J. Am. Diet. Assoc. 73:48.

Grant-Whiting, M., and R. M. Leverton. 1960. Reliability of dietary appraisal. Comparison between laboratory analysis and calculation from tables of food values. Am. J. Public Health 50:815.

Gray, C. E., and N. R. Blackman. 1947. More high school student diets evaluated. J. Home Econ. 39:505.

Groover, M. E., Jr., L. Boone, P. C. Houk, and S. Wolf. 1967. Problems in quantitation of dietary survey. J. Am. Med. Assoc. 201:86.

Grossman, E., and D. Popka. 1976. Methodology of a household food consumption survey in Cincinnati, Ohio, Nov. 1969–Jan. 1970. Unpublished.

Guggenham, K., J. Ilan, T. Vogo, and G. Mindel. 1960. Nutritional status and food consumption of pregnant women in a development area of Israel. Br. J. Nutr. 14:347.

Guthrie, H. A. 1963. Nutritional intake of infants. J. Am. Diet. Assoc. 43:120.

Hankin, J. H., and R. Huenemann. 1967. A short dietary method for epidemiologic studies. I. Developing standard methods for interpreting seven-day measured food records. J. Am. Diet. Assoc. 50:487.

Hankin, J. H., W. E. Reynolds, and S. Margen. 1967. A short dietary method for epidemiologic studies. II. Variability of measured nutrient intakes. Am. J. Clin. Nutr. 20:935.

Hankin, J. H., R. A. Stallones, and H. B. Messenger. 1968. A short dietary method for epidemiologic studies. III. Development of questionnaire. Am. J. Epidemiol. 87:285.

Hankin, J. H., H. B. Messenger, and R. A. Stallones. 1970. A short dietary method for epidemiologic studies. IV. Evaluation of questionnaire. Am. J. Epidemiol. 91:562.

Hankin, J. H., G. G. Rhoads, and G. A. Glober. 1975. A dietary method for epidemiologic study of gastrointestinal cancer. Am. J. Clin. Nutr. 28:1055–1061.

Hankin, J. H., M. S. Rawlings, and A. Nomura. 1978. Assessment of a short dietary method for a prospective study on cancer. Am. J. Clin. Nutr. 31:355.

Heady, J. A. 1961. Diets of bank clerks. Development of a method of classifying the diets of individuals for use in epidemiological studies. J. R. Stat. Soc. Ser. A (Gen.) 125:336.

Hiemstra, S. 1968. Food consumption, prices, expenditures. U.S. Dep. Agric., Econ. Res. Serv. Agric. Econ. Dep. Rep. 138. 193 pp.

Huenemann, R., and D. Turner. 1942. Methods of dietary investigation. J. Am. Diet. Assoc. 18:562.

Huenemann, R. L., F. E. French, and J. M. Bierman. 1961. Diets of pregnant women in Kauai, Hawaii. J. Am. Diet. Assoc. 39:567.

Hummel, F. C., *et al.* 1942. Chemical composition of twenty-two common foods and comparison of analytical and calculated values of diets. J. Nutr. 24:41.

Hunter, G., J. Kastetic, and M. Ball. 1948. Assessment of diets: Analysis versus computation from food tables. Can. J. Res. Sec. E 26:367.

ICNND. Manual for nutrition surveys, 2nd ed. 1963. U.S. Government Printing Office, Washington, D.C. Chap. VII, Dietary studies, pp. 159–230 and 249–260.

Kaser, M., *et al.* 1947. A comparison of the calculated and determined caloric and vitamin content of mixed diets. Am. J. Hyg. 46:297.

Keys, A. 1968. Dietary survey methods. *In* den Hartog, C., K. Buzina, F. Fidanza, A. Keys, and P. Roine, eds. Studies of cardiovascular epidemiology of heart disease. M. Wyt & Sons, Rotterdam. Pp. 9–29.

Keys, A. 1979. Dietary survey methods. *In* R. Levy, B. Rifkind, B. Dennis, and N. Ernst, eds. Nutrition, lipids, and coronary heart disease. Raven Press, New York, Pp. 1–23.

Koehne, M. 1935. Probable accuracy of dietary studies. J. Am. Diet. Assoc. 11:105.

LeBovit, C., and D. Baker. 1965. Food consumption and dietary levels of older households in Rochester, New York. U.S. Dep. Agric. Home Econ. Res. Rep. 25. 91 pp.

Lechtig, A., C. Yarbrough, R. Martorell, H. Delgado, and R. D. Klein. 1976. The one day recall dietary survey: A review of its usefulness to estimate protein and calorie intake. Arch. Latinoam. Nutr. 26:1243.

Leitch, I., and F. C. Aitken. 1949. Technique and interpretations of dietary surveys. Nutr. Abst. Rev. 19:507.

Leverton, R. 1937. A comparison of values obtained by calculation and by analysis for iron content of 85 mixed diets. J. Am. Diet. Assoc. 13:139.

Leverton, R. M., and A. G. Marsh. 1939. Comparison of food intakes for weekdays and for Saturday and Sunday. J. Home Econ. 31:111.

Leverton, R. M., and J. Pazur. 1957. Food practices and nutritional status of typical Nebraska families. Nebr. Univ. Agric. Exp. Stn. Misc. Publ. 5. 52 pp.

Linusson, E. E., D. Sanjur, and E. C. Erickson. 1974. Validating the 24-hour recall method as a dietary survey tool. Arch. Latinoam. Nutr. 24:277.

Lockhart. E. E., *et al.* 1944. Study of nutritional quality of dietaries by chemical analysis. J. Am. Diet. Assoc. 20:742.

Madden, J. P., S. J. Goodman, and H. A. Guthrie. 1976. Validity of the 24-hr. recall. Analysis of data obtained from elderly subjects. J. Am. Diet. Assoc. 68:143.

Majonner, L., and Y. Hall. 1968. The national diet heart study—assessment of dietary adherence. J. Am. Diet. Assoc. 52:288.

Manalo, R., and J. Jones. 1966. The content of constant diets: A comparison between analyzed and calculated values. Am. J. Clin. Nutr. 18:339.

Mann, G., G. Pearson, T. Gordon, and T. Dawber. 1962. Diet and cardiovascular disease in the Framingham study. I. Measurement of dietary intake. Am. J. Clin. Nutr. 11:200.

Marr, J. W. 1971. Individual dietary surveys: Purposes and methods. World Rev. Nutr. Diet. 13:105.

Marr, J. W. 1973. Dietary survey methods. *In* Individual and group aspects. Proc. R. Soc. Med. 66:639.

Marr, J. W., J. A. Heady, and J. N. Morris. 1961. Towards a method for large-scale individual diet surveys. Pages 85–91 *in* Proc. 3rd Int. Congr. Dietet. Newman Books, London.

McCann, M. B., M. F. Trulson, and F. J. Stare. 1961. Follow-up study of serum cholesterol, diet and physical findings of Italian-American factory workers. Am. J. Clin. Nutr. 9:351.

McCay, C. M., *et al.* 1945. Nutritive value of food served in some large Navy messes. J. Am. Diet. Assoc. 21:88.

McHenry, E. W., H. P. Ferguson, and J. Gurland. 1945. Sources of errors in dietary surveys. Can. J. Public Health 36:355.

Meredith, A., A. Matthews, M. Zickefoose, *et al.* 1951. How well do school children recall what they have eaten? J. Am. Diet. Assoc. 27:749.

Mickelsen, O., *et al.* 1947. The determination of fat and its relation to the calculated caloric value of diets. J. Am. Diet. Assoc. 23:952.

Ministry of Agriculture, Fisheries and Food, National Food Survey Committee. 1972. Household food consumptions and expenditures. Her Majesty's Stationery Office, London. 218 pp.

Mongeau, E. 1974. Dietary assessment of nutritional status. The assessment of nutritional status, Proc. Miles Symp., June 25, 1973. Saskatchewan University, Canada.

Moore, M. C., B. C. Judlin, and P. McA. Kennemur. 1967. Using graduated food models in taking dietary histories. J. Am. Diet. Assoc. 51:447.

Morgan, A. F., ed. 1959. Nutritional status. Calif. Agric. Exp. Stn. Bull. 769. 131 pp.

Morris, J. N. 1970. Uses of epidemiology. Livingstone, Edinburgh.

Morrison, S. D., C. F. Russell, and J. Stevenson. 1949. Estimating food intake by questioning and weighing: A one day survey of eight subjects. Br. J. Nutr. 3:V.

Murray, J. 1970. USDA food consumption surveys—A historical review with special reference to the development and testing of collection methods. Unpublished.

Norris, T. 1949. Dietary surveys: Their technique and interpretation. FAO Nutritional Studies No. 4, Washington, D.C., December 1949. 108 pp.

Ohlson, M. A., L. Jackson, J. Boek, *et al.* 1950. Nutrition and dietary habits of aging women. Am. J. Public Health 40:1101.

Owen, G., P. Garry, K. Kram, *et al.* 1969. Nutritional status of preschool children. A pilot study. Am. J. Clin. Nutr. 22:1444.

Owen, G., K. M. Kram, P. J. Garry, *et al.* 1974. A study of nutritional status of preschool children in the United States, 1968–70. Pediatrics 53(Pt. II, Suppl.):597.

Pao, E. M., and M. C. Burk. 1975. Portion sizes and day's intakes of selected foods. U.S. Dep. Agric. ARS-NE-67. 70 pp.

Patterson, L. 1971. Dietary intake and physical development of Phoenix area children. J. Am. Diet. Assoc. 59:106.

Patterson, J. M., and E. W. McHenry. 1941. Errors with calculation of the nutritive value of food intake. I. Comparison of calculated and determined amounts of calories, protein and fat. Can. J. Public Health 32:362.

Paul, O., M. H. Lepper, W. H. Phelan, *et al.* 1963. A longitudinal study of coronary heart disease. Circulation 28:20.

Pekkarinen, M. 1970. Methodology in the collection of food consumption data. World Rev. Nutr. Diet. 12:145.

Pekkarinen, M., S. Kivioja, and L. Jortikka. 1967. A comparison of the food intake of rural families estimated by a one-day recall and precise weighing method. Voeding 28:470.

Pekkarinen, M., S. Kivioja, and L. Jortikka. 1968. A comparison of the food intake of rural families estimated by one-day recall and precise weighing methods. *In* C. den Hartog, K. Buzina, F. Fidanza, A. Keys, and P. Roine, eds. Dietary studies and epidemiology of heart diseases. M. Wyt & Sons, Rotterdam, The Hague.

Pilcher, H. L., J. M. Leichseming, S. P. Frommes, and L. M. Norris. 1961. Comparison of analyzed and calculated energy values of food intakes of adult women. Metabolism 10:475.

Proceedings of Conference on Methods for Evaluating Nutritional Status of Mothers, Infants and Children. 1947. Res. Lab. Children's Fund of Michigan, Detroit. 93 pp. Mimeo.

Quackenbush, G. G., and J. D. Shaffer. 1960. Collecting food purchase data by Consumer Panel—A methodological report on MSU Consumer Panel, 1951–58. Mich. State Univ. Agric. Exp. Stn. Tech. Bull. 279. 73 pp.

Reagan, B., and E. Grossman. 1951. Rural levels of living in Lee and Jones Counties, Mississippi, 1945 and a comparison of two methods of data collection. U. S. Dep. Agric. Inform. Bull. 41. 164 pp.

Reddy, S. 1968. Practical problems in obtaining valid and reliable information on household food utilization. J. Trop. Pediatr. 14:66.

Reed, R. B., and B. S. Burke. 1954. Collection and analysis of dietary intake data. Am. J. Public Health 44:1015.

Reshef, A., and L. Epstein. 1972. Reliability of a dietary questionnaire. Am. J. Clin. Nutr. 25:91.

Response Analysis Corporation. 1976. Report of findings food methodology study. Prepared for Consumer and Food Economics Institute, U. S. Department of Agriculture, Hyattsville, Md.

Roberts, L. J., and M. Waite. 1925. A dietary study made in a day nursery by the individual method. J. Home Econ. 17:80;142.

Roine, P., and M. Pekkarinen. 1968. Methodology of dietary surveys. Int. Z. Vitaminforch. 11:31.

Samuelson, G. 1970. An epidemiological study of child health and nutrition in a northern Swedish county. II. Methodological study of the recall technique. Nutr. Metab. 12:321.

Samuelson, G. 1971. An epidemiological study of child health and nutrition in a northern Swedish county. I. Food consumption survey. Acta Paediatr. Scand. Suppl. 214. 44 pp.

Schaefer, A. E. 1966. Assessment of nutritional status: Food intake studies. Page 217 *in* G. H. Beaton and E. W. McHenry, eds. Nutrition: A comprehensive treatise, Vol. III., Chap. 6, Academic Press, New York.

Semmons, E. M., and E. W. McHenry. 1944. Errors in the calculation of the nutritive value of food intake. IV. Comparison of calculated and determined amounts of calcium. Can. J. Public Health 34:286.

Sprauve, M. E., and M. L. Dodds. 1965. Dietary survey of adolescents in the Virgin Islands. J. Am. Diet. Assoc. 47:287.

Stead, R. M. 1968. Assessment of methods of dietary appraisal. A comparison of two different modifications of Burke's dietary history method. S. Afr. Med. J. 42:961.

Steele, B. F., and R. D. Tucker. 1952. Influence of dietary interpretations as calculated nutritive value of the diet. Page 78 *in* C. M. Young, *et al.* Cooperative nutritional status studies in the Northeast Region. III. Dietary methodology studies. Univ. Mass. Agric. Exp. Stn. Bull. No. 469.

Steele, B. F., R. E. Franklin, V. L. Smudski, and C. M. Young. 1951. Use of checked seven-day records in a dietary survey. J. Am. Diet. Assoc. 27:957.

Steele, B. F., V. L. Smudski, R. E. Franklin, and C. M. Young. 1952. Comparison between three methods of assessing nutrient intake of children. Page 59 *in* C. M. Young, *et al.* Cooperative nutritional status studies in the Northeast Region. III. Dietary methodology studies. Univ. Mass. Agric. Exp. Stn. Bull. No. 469.

Stefanik, P. A., and M. F. Trulson. 1962. Determining the frequency intakes of foods in large group studies. Am. J. Clin. Nutr. 11:335.

Stefferud, A., ed. 1959. Food: The yearbook of agriculture, 1959. U.S. Government Printing Office, Washington, D.C.

Stevens, H., R. Bleiler, and M. Ohlson. 1963. Dietary intake of five groups of subjects. J. Am. Diet. Assoc. 42:387.

Stock, A. L., and E. F. Wheeler. 1972. Evaluation of meals cooked by large-scale methods: A comparison of chemical analysis and calculation from food tables. Br. J. Nutr. 27:439.

Strong, J. A., and R. Passmore. 1967. Adaption to overfeeding in man. Proc. Nutr. Soc. 26:163.

Sudman, S., and R. Ferber. 1971. Experiments in obtaining consumer expenditures by diary methods. Am. Stat. Assoc. J. 66(336):725–735.

Swanson, P., E. W. Willis, E. Jebe, *et al.* 1959. Food intakes of 2,189 women in five north central states. Iowa State Coll., Iowa Agric. Home Econ. Exp. Stn. Res. Bull. 468. Pp. 476–499.

Symposium—American Dietetic Association. 1951–1952. Dietary study methods, October 1950. J. Am. Diet. Assoc. 27:558, 745, 838, 968; 28:43.

Symposium—American Institute of Nutrition. 1950. Symposium on Nutritional Appraisal of Human Subjects, Atlantic City, April 20, 1950. Maynard, L. A. Evaluation of dietary survey methods. Fed. Proc. 9:598.

Symposium—American Public Health Association. 1960–1961. Methodology for dietary studies in epidemiological surveys, 1959. Am. J. Public Health 50:803, 815, 824; 51:70.

Symposium on Recent Advances in the Appraisal of the Nutrient Intake and Nutritional Status of Man. 1962. MIT, Boston, March 1962. Am. J. Clin. Nutr. 11:335–404.

Tasker, J., *et al.* 1967. Dietary survey by weighment method—A comparison of random day, 3-day and 7-day period. Indian J. Med. Res. 55:90.

Taylor, E.C. 1970. The impact of computer analysis on the design of dietary surveys. Proc. Nutr. Soc. 29:135.

Third International Congress of Dietetics Proceedings. 1961. Wm. Byles & Sons, Ltd., Bradford, Yorkshire, England.

Thomas, R. V., *et al.* 1950a. Nutritional status of children. XII. Evaluation by computing the food intake of a group and by weighing and analyzing food eaten by representative subjects. J. Am. Diet. Assoc. 26:788.

Thomas, R. V., M. Rutledge, E. Beach, *et al.* 1950b. Nutritional status of children. XIII. Accuracy of calculated intakes of food components with respect to analytical values. J. Am. Diet. Assoc. 26:889.

Thomson, A. M. 1958. Diet in pregnancy. 1. Dietary survey technique and the nutritive value of diets taken by primigravidae. Br. J. Nutr. 12:446.

Tinsley, W. V. 1947. Development of instruments for evaluating food practices, nutrition information, and school lunch programs and their use in nutrition education at the elementary level. Doctor's thesis, Univ. of Minn., St. Paul. 333 pp. (Abstr. in J. Home Econ. 41:514, 1949.)

Toscani, V. 1948. Comparison of analyzed with calculated diets. Food Res. 13:187.

Trulson, M. F. 1951. Assessment of methods of dietary intake. Synopsis from Ph.D. thesis. Mimeo to author.

Trulson, M. F. 1954. Assessment of dietary study methods. I. Comparison of methods for obtaining data for clinical work. J. Am. Diet. Assoc. 30:991.

Trulson, M.F. 1955. Assessment of dietary study methods. II. Variability of eating practices and determination of sample size and duration of dietary surveys. J. Am. Diet. Assoc. 31:797.

Trulson, M. F. 1960a. Report of Diet Methodology Committee. *In* Conference on Methodology in Epidemiological Studies in Cardiovascular Disease, Princeton, N.J., April 24–26, 1959. Am. J. Public Health Suppl. 50. 124 pp.

Trulson, M. F. 1960b. Subcommittee on Methodology for Diet Appraisal. Pages 39–52 *in* Conference on Methodology in Epidemiological Studies in Cardiovascular Disease, Princeton, N.J., April 24–26, 1959. Am. J. Public Health Suppl. 50: October 1960.

Trulson, M. F., and M. B. McCann. 1959. Comparison of dietary survey methods. J. Am. Diet. Assoc. 35:672.

U.S. Department of Agriculture, Agricultural Research Service. 1972a. Food and nutrient intake of individuals in the United States, spring 1965. U.S. Dep. Agric. Household Food Consumption Survey, 1965–66, Rep. No. 11. 289 pp.

U.S. Department of Agriculture, Agricultural Research Service. 1972b. Food consumption of households in the United States, seasons and year, 1965–66. U.S. Dep. Agric. Household Food Consumption Survey, 1965–66. Rep. No. 12. 217 pp.

U.S. Department of Health, Education, and Welfare, Health Services and Mental Health Administration, Center for Disease Control. 1972. Ten-state survey, 1968–70. DHEW Publ. No. (HSM) 72-8133. 340 pp.

Van Schaik, Th. F. S. M. 1968. Practical problems in estimating dietary intake at home. Int. Z. Vitaminforsch. 11:43.

Viteri, F., and B. Torim. 1975. Ingestion calorica y trahajo fisico de obreros agricos en Guatemala. Effect de la suplementacion alimentaria y su lagar en los programos de salud. Bol. Of. San. Pan. 78:58.

Wait, B., and L. J. Roberts. 1932. Studies in the food requirement of adolescent girls. II. Daily food requirements in the energy intake of the individual. J. Am. Diet. Assoc. 8:323.

Wakefield, L. N. 1966. The interview technique in research—Sources of bias. J. Home Econ. 58:640.

Walberg, S., and W. Adams. 1965. Calculated and determined values in constant diets. J. Am. Diet. Assoc. 47:37.

Wertz, A. W., M. E. Lojkin, E. H. Morse, *et al.* 1952. Comparison of determined and calculated amounts of eight nutrients in one day's food intake of twenty-one subjects. *In* C. M. Young, *et al.* Cooperative nutritional status studies in the Northeast Region. III. Contributions to dietary methodology studies. Univ. Mass. Agric. Exp. Stn. Bull. No. 469.

White, H. S. 1969. Inorganic elements in weighed diets of girls and young women. J. Am. Diet. Assoc. 55:38.

Widdowson, E. M. 1947. A study of individual children's diets. Med. Res. Counc. Spec. Rep. Ser. No. 257. His Majesty's Stationery Office, London. 196 pp.

Widdowson, E. M., and R. A. McCance. 1943. Food tables: Their scope and limitations. Lancet 1:230.

Wiehl, D. G., and R. Reed. 1960. Development of new or improved dietary methods for epidemiological investigations. Am. J. Public Health 50:824.

Youland, D. M., *et al.* 1976. Practices and problems in HANES. Dietary data methodology. J. Am. Diet. Assoc. 68:22.

Young, C. M. 1965. Comparison of results of dietary surveys made by different methods. Pages 119–126 *in* New horizons in dietetics. Proc. 4th Int. Congr. Dietet. Ivar Hoeggstrom Tryckeri AB, Stockholm.

Young, C. M., and E. W. McHenry. 1942–1943. Errors in the calculation of the nutritive value of food intake. II. Comparison of calculated and determined amounts of ascorbic acid. III. Comparison of calculated and determined amounts of iron. Can. J. Public Health 33:224, 34:367.

Young, C. M., and K. Musgrave. 1951. The use of the dietary scorecard. J. Am. Diet. Assoc. 27:745.

Young, C. M., *et al.* 1951a. Nutritional status survey, Groton Township, New York. II. Nutrient usage of families and individuals. J. Am. Diet. Assoc. 26:776.

Young, C. M., V. Smudski, and B. Steele. 1951b. Fall and spring diets in school children in New York State. J. Am. Diet. Assoc. 27:289.

Young, C. M., F. W. Chalmers, H. N. Church, *et al.* 1952a. A comparison of dietary study methods. I. Dietary history vs. seven-day record. J. Am. Diet. Assoc. 28:124.

Young, C. M., G. C. Hagan, R. E. Tucker, and W. D. Foster. 1952b. A comparison of dietary study methods. II. Dietary history vs. seven-day record vs. 24-hour recall. J. Am. Diet. Assoc. 28:218.

Young, C. M., *et al.* 1952c. Cooperative nutritional status studies in the Northeast Region. III. Contributions to dietary methodology studies. Univ. Mass. Agric. Exp. Stn. Bull. No. 469, Amherst. 95 pp.

Young, C. M., F. Chalmers, H. Church, *et al.* 1953a. Subject's estimation of food intake and calculated nutritive value of the diet. J. Am. Diet. Assoc. 29:1216.

Young, C. M., R. Franklin, W. Foster, and B. Steele. 1953b. Weekly variation in nutrient intake of young adults. J. Am. Diet. Assoc. 29:459.

Yudkin, J. 1951. Dietary surveys: Variation in weekly intake of nutrients. Br. J. Nutr. 5:177.

Yudkin, J., and J. Roddy. 1966. Assessment of sugar intake: Validity of the questionnaire method. Br. J. Nutr. 20:807.

Ziffer, H., O. Frank, G. Christakis, *et al.* 1967. Data analysis strategy for nutritional surveys of 642 New York City school children. Am. J. Clin. Nutr. 20:858.

Mail Diary Method for Collecting Food Purchasing and Food Usage Information from Consumer Panels

I. J. ABRAMS

INTRODUCTION

The Market Research Corporation of American (MRCA) has specialized in collecting information from large samples on household purchases of grocery products, textile products, and other frequently bought consumer products using the mail diary techniques. Similarly, it has collected detail information on household food preparation and on individual food intake.

The National Consumer Panel (NCP) consists of a nationally distributed sample of 7,500 households, reporting every week in a printed diary their purchases of selected foods and other grocery products, on a continuing basis for extended periods of time. The National Household Menu Census (MC) Study, usually conducted every 5 years, is based on a subsample of 4,000 households selected from the NCP. Each study spans a period of 12 months, in which each household reports for 14 consecutive days all food preparation and consumption at home and away from home, using separate daily diaries.

The NCP has been operating commerically since 1942, and the Menu Census Service has been repeated each 5 years since 1957, including an interim one-half sample size study conducted in 1975. These two services are designed to satisfy the information requirements of food-processing and marketing companies and of their advertising agencies. Reports are sold on a syndicated basis, whereby the costs are shared by the multiple users of the same information.

THE NATIONAL CONSUMER PANEL

Objectives

NCP measures the end of the food distribution channel, where the product enters the home of the consumer. It thus identifies who buys the product, how often, at what price, and from which store. Since these measurements are made continuously over time, NCP is able to identify all the competing brands, forms, and other product variations that are available to the consumer in a given food category and the switching patterns that consumers make in purchase choices among the different brands over time. The data from NCP are usually summarized on a monthly and quarterly cycle, with special analyses performed on a semiannual or an annual basis. The data are used to track consumer purchases in a product category over time; to evaluate the effectiveness of various marketing, promotion, advertising, and pricing strategies employed by the client or by its competitors; to monitor the "life cycle" of various brands or products; to evaluate new entries into the market; to spot target segments exhibiting special consumer preferences; to identify opportunities for new products; to evaluate potential acquisitions of individual brands or of food manfacturing companies; and in general to provide a continuously updated data base suitable for diagnosing problems encountered in the market place, devising solutions to these problems, and methods of evaluating the success of such solutions.

The essential characteristic of these data is that they are collected longitudinally from a large sample of individual households, on a frequent basis, for predefined produce categories, on a sufficient detail basis to identify brands, types, subtypes, forms, packages, package sizes, individual prices paid by the consumers, the use of coupons or other purchase incentives, and the identity of the stores from which the purchases were made. Of course, this information represents consumption by the entire household and is not usually broken down by each individual member of that household, except in special cases. In this respect, the information is still at an aggregate level, and not at the individual eater level.

Sample Design and Maintenance

The basic design of NCP is a stratified probability sample, incorporating 440 primary sample units. These consist of about 220 different locations representing all large cities, most of the intermediate-size cities, and samples from the smaller cities, rural communities, and farm areas. Most of these geographical areas are then divided into two cells, representing small versus large households. Since the sample is operated continuously over time, the main function of this cell structure is to provide a framework for maintaining the balance of the sample to the population and to control all replacement recruiting efforts. This maintenance or replacement recruiting is purposive in nature and usually consists of replacing a lost household with another one living in the same area and having similar demographic characteristics. Households that move from their original area are maintained in the sample and when necessary are later replaced by new households that live in the area to which they moved. Thus, NCP continues to diffuse across the entire United States from its primary sampling unit. In fact, its distribution anticipates the results that are later obtained through updates in the U.S. Census. Recruiting of replacement households is done in several ways. The more frequent method is by mail, using telephone lists. Personal interviewing may be used when the need arises to replace special kinds of households. At times, telephone recruiting may be used. Since it is usually difficult to recruit newly formed young households, NCP resorts to recruiting children of existing panel members when they leave home and set up their own households. NCP does not accept volunteers or references provided by current panel members.

Recruited households are trained for a period of from 1 to 3 months prior to their inclusion in the production sample. During that period, their weekly diaries are examined carefully for accuracy and completeness of recording, and write-backs to the households are used to inform them of any errors or misinterpretation of instructions.

Compensation

Reporting households are compensated with a variable schedule of "points," which are redeemable for gifts through a premium catalog, similar to green stamps or other such saving stamps. A nominal number of points is given for returning a diary, whether on time or late, regardless of whether any purchases are reported in it. Bonuses are given for prompt reporting and for returning all diaries in the month. Periodically, NCP households receive additional questionnaires, and once a year they receive the basic Household Classification Questionnaire. Additional points are always given for such supplementary questionnaires. A special effort is made to encourage the continuity of panel membership of hard-to-keep young households by providing gifts at the birthdates of small children.

Weekly Diaries and Other Questionnaires

The weekly diary has been recently redesigned to permit tearing out and returning only pages in which the household reported purchases of specified products. This is an effort to control the mail costs, which constitutes a significant portion of the operations cost of a weekly diary. The front cover of the diary captures from the household information on every trip to any store that sells products contained in the diary. Households are encouraged to record each trip as soon as it is completed, in order to remind the household to report purchases of products contained in the diary. The date and identity of the stores is reported only on the face of the diary, and the sequential number of the store trip is then reported on the first column of each entry. A standard entry inside the diary provides space for reporting the brand of the specific product; some product details unique to that category; the number of packages purchased; the size of each package; the unit or total price paid; and any special coupons, discounts, or store deals.

Great care is exercised in the description of the products to be reported, through examples provided to further describe that product within various check boxes for that entry, through the description of other characteristics of the purchase, and in the positioning of each diary section in relation to other sections on that page and on other pages of the diary. When new sections are added to the diary, they are usually printed on the bottom half of the front cover, in order to bring their attention to the panel members, and later the section is inserted into an appropriate location within the diary. Changes in the positions of various items in the diary are made very infrequently, so that households are able to remember the locations of most products that must be entered, and thus reduce the total effort required in maintaining such diaries. A detailed Index of Products to be entered is printed on the inside front cover of the diary, to help the reporter find the location where to enter a specific item, as well as to inform the reporter whether or not a specific product should be reported in the diary.

Frozen and refrigerated products are positioned in the early pages of the diary, since they are usually unpacked and stored first when the household returns from a shopping trip, followed by shelf stable canned and packaged products, and concluded with household and personal care products. Space is provided for entering purchases that cannot fit in the space allocated in the body of the diary and also occasionally for reporting products that could be entered in one of several places, but which the household is not sure where to report. Space is also provided at the end for reporting changes in the composition of the household that week.

The Household Classification Questionnaire is administered each April to all NCP households. A similar form is also completed by each household when it is recruited. Detail information is reported on the income, education, and other demographic characteristics of each household member; and information on ownership of several appliances, on the type of residence, and on other characteristics that are required for classifying the household into the many categories that are used by manufacturers and by advertising agencies for analyzing patterns of household food purchasing. It is, of course, also used in balancing the sample to the population. Even though the questionnaire contains several sensitive personal items such as income, age, and the like, almost all households report this information on a regular basis.

Occasionally a custom or temporary test market panel is recruited in locations specified by the client, where a new product is being tested by the manufacturer or by its competitors. Households for that market are recruited independently of NCP and are maintained for a limited period of time, usually from 6 to 18 months. They report in a very small diary, which contains, in addition to the product category of interest, several other categories, whose functions are to mask the desired category, and thereby prevent overstimulating the panel members to purchase or explore items under test. Households that complete their test panel assignments may later be recruited into the National Consumer Panel if it is deficient in these kinds of households in the particular market.

Data Transcription and Editing

All entries in those diary sections that are currently sold are transcribed by coders for machine processing. The diary sections are formatted to collect specific product characteristics that are needed by the client, and code structures are devised to capture this information in a unique way. Since all purchases of the specified category are reported by panel members, regardless of what region of the country they live in, and from which store or outlet they purchased the item, including home deliveries, door-to-door salesman, mail order, home grown or canned, etc., the code structures are frequently extensive and detailed. They are continuously updated as new products or variations of existing products are reported by household members. These code structures also include information on known package sizes by brands, price ranges, outlets in which specific brands may be obtained, such as private label, and the like, and this information is then used to machine edit the transcribed information. All errors are returned to the coding department for verification or correction, and occasionally require follow-up with the reporting households.

The diaries are usually mailed back on the Sunday or Monday following the reporting week, and most diaries are received by us by the following Friday. The entries are transcribed and checked by the end of the second week following the reporting week, at which time "flash" reports can be produced if needed. Reports are produced for two 4-week months, followed by a 5-week month each quarter. The quarters consist of 13 weeks each, adding up to a 52-week year. For some clients, the reporting is made each

4-week month, or each 12-week quarter, resulting in 13 monthly reports per year, synchronized with the reporting cycle of SAMI.

Reports

Monthly and quarterly reports are usually delivered to clients 2 to 3 weeks following the close of the data period covered in these reports. Monthly and quarterly reports contain brand shares based on pounds or packages bought by households during the reporting period, projected to regions and U.S. totals; the number and percent of households who bought the product at least once during the time periods; the average frequency of purchasing occasions of each item; the average price paid; the average price paid when the purchase was on a special deal or store sale; the average quantity per buying household; the average size of a purchase; and other similar "buyer" statistics. Special reports frequently include statistics on share of total household requirements that were satisfied by each key product type or brand; percent of households who repeated purchasing the brand from the previous quarter or the previous year; and the amount of purchases of a particular category that were switched from one brand to another over two time periods.

A substantial repertoire of special studies has been developed for processing longitudinal consumer purchase information, in order to address unique problems that manufacturers encounter in the market place. Some of these analytical techniques are designed to identify target populations of "heavy users," or "loyal buyers of a brand," or "promising potential buyers" of a particular brand or type. Special attention has been devoted to predicting the rate of adoption of a new product in the market, and ultimate success or failure of a new product, and the level that it may attain in the second or third year following its introduction, based on as short an observation period as possible.

Validity and Accuracy of the Data

NCP and test panels are based on samples of "Households" following U.S. Census definitions. They usually exclude persons living in institutions, such as schools, dormitories, hospitals, residence hotels, and the armed forces. They do include households composed of single individuals, or of unrelated individuals sharing a common housing unit. Therefore, information reported by these panels is representative only of food purchases made by the corresponding household segment of the population. This excludes about 5 percent of the population.

Since all reporting is done by mail and in writing, the samples exclude households that are illiterate, or those containing no potential reporter who writes and reads English. Also, since recruiting is frequently done from mailing lists extracted from telephone directories, the sample tends to be deficient in households that do not own telephones.

In general, the projected sample is reasonably well balanced to U.S. Census on most key demographic characteristics. Since panel members have to be willing to report their purchases of a large number of product categories on a weekly basis, over extended periods of time, the sample will tend to have very few members in which the homemaker, or other potential reporter, is unwilling to undertake such a task. The willingness to do this work is, in a broad sense, correlated with the interest of the homemaker in the task of purchasing foods, or in other aspects related to maintaining a home, to shopping, and to reporting on such activities. Although the sample has representative members from every strata of the population, cooperation is lowest among single young persons, mothers with small children, persons with very low income, and especially those living in central cities. By contrast, households in middle-income-class suburbia, or with a full-time homemaker, tend to cooperate more readily when recruited, and then tend to stay in the panel for much longer periods of time. Incentives for cooperation vary widely and are not necessarily related to the level of compensation for this work. Of course, many homemakers consider the gifts that they get through cooperation to be "independently earned income." Some homemakers view cooperation as a method of influencing manufacturers to produce the kind of products they prefer.

On the whole, data projected from NCP match reasonably well levels and trends of purchases known from independent sources. However, some products suffer from some degree of undercoverage, which may be caused in part by a forgetfulness of the panel members to report all purchases of the product and in part from underpurchasing by panel members of a specific product because it is, in the eyes of a more skilled or experienced or knowledgeable consumer, more expensive or less economical. Underreporting can occasionally result from imprecise or ambiguous format and description of a product in the diary. This may occur especially for products whose food category is ambiguous and that actually do not belong clearly to any specific category. In fact, manufacturers try to identify new product categories and market new products, which do not have to compete with well-established brands. It is therefore necessary at times to experiment in the way the item is described in the diary before panel households learn to report the item properly. Similarly, overcoverage may occur because panel cooperators tend to buy the more economical sizes, or the brands that offer more value for the money, or to redeem coupons and buy items on sale more often, and the like. However, because these tendencies are relatively constant over time, their main effect may be on the level of the projected data, but not as much on trends and other aspects of the information being collected. Because a great deal is known about these biases in the data, it is possible to anticipate them and to account for them in producing continuing or special studies.

The accuracy of any item of information depends to a large part on the degree of variability in purchase patterns from one household to the next, and therefore on the size of the sample and on the percent of households who regularly buy that item. The smaller the number of households buying the item, the higher the variability in the computed average amount per buying household. Since the number of households buying any particular item increases for longer time periods, it is therefore occasionally possible to obtain the desired level of accuracy in an estimated purchase incidence of frequency for a brand at a semiannual or an annual level, when it is too small on a monthly or quarterly basis. When additional accuracy is required for a monthly or a quarterly time period in a given area, it is occasionally possible to augment the NCP in a particular region by adding "test panel" households to the sample. In general, the size of test market panels is usually determined by the level of accuracy that is needed in the reported information.

THE NATIONAL HOUSEHOLD MENU CENSUS SERVICE

Objectives

The Menu Census Service is designed to collect detail information on the ultimate disposition of all food products in terms of their consumption by individuals as obtained, or their use in preparation of other dishes to be eaten by individuals. In this respect, the Menu Census observes the true end of the food distribution system from the farm to its final use. From the point of view of food intake by individuals, information collected by the National Consumer Panel still represents an aggregate measurement at that point in the distribution system where the in-home inventory is replenished. This in-home inventory can be substantial, and foods may remain there for extended periods of time. Although liquid milk, fresh meat, bread, and similar perishable products are generally consumed within a few days from their entry into the home, others, such as powdered milk, canned soup, spices and seasonings, dehydrated vegetables, instant mixes, and the like, are frequently stocked by the household for weeks, months, or even years after purchase, and are thus further removed from individual eating.

Some of the primary uses of data collected in the Menu Census Studies are: (a) Early identification of trends in food usage by type, form, packaging, etc., which may lead to new product innovation, product modifications, new marketing strategies applied to existing products, new advertising approaches, and the like. (b) A better understanding of the way specific products or forms of a product are used or served by household or by individuals, leading to the identification of population segments with special needs, and thus suggesting more effective marketing or advertising techniques, or to modifications of the form or the packaging of the product. (c) A determination of the customer base of a given food category, leading to a decision to enter that market, or to acquire an existing manufacturer or brand in the market, or to discontinue participation in that category. (d) More recently, the Menu Census has been used to evaluate the exposure of individuals, by various age-groups, or by other characteristics, to specific food additives from the diet, in connection with regulatory activities of various governmental agencies, such as FDA, FTC, USDA, and others; the data have been used by FDA and the National Academy of Sciences to compute individual intake of food additives in the GRAS survey, PHASE II, and are currently being used in the PHASE III survey. (e) The data have been used by FDA for ad hoc studies of the exposure of individuals to various direct or indirect additives to foods; they have similarly been used by commercial clients to evaluate the levels of exposure of individuals to alternate food additives, such as sweeteners, colorings, flavorings, and the like, in the search for a replacement to a currently used substance whose continued use may later be restricted. (f) They have been used to define foods that belong to selected categories or subcategories, in terms of their substitutability, in judicial hearings involving two competing manufacturers, or involving the government and a manufacturer. (g) They have been used to evaluate the nutritional contributions of groups of specific foods, or of meals containing specific foods, or of the dietary status of individuals with differing food consumption patterns.

Sample Design, Recruiting, Training, Daily Diary and Other Forms, Compensation

The Menu Census is usually conducted once in 5 years, from July through the following June. It was begun in July 1957, and the last study was completed in June 1978. An interim study was also conducted during the calendar year of 1975. Each study consists of 4,000 households, selected from the NCP, including whenever possible only households that reported in NCP for at least 6 months. The 1975 interim study contained only 2,000 households, most of whom were drawn from the previous Fourth Menu Census Study, which was conducted during July 1972 through June 1973. Table 1 shows a comparison between the demographics of the Sixth Menu Census sample and the U.S. Census.

Each household reports all food preparation and consumption at home and

TABLE 1 Sixth National Household Menu Census, Composition of the Sample, Annual Summary, July 1977–June 1978

	Households and Household Members Distributed by Demographic Characteristics				
	Households in Sample		Persons in Sample		U.S. Census Households
Household Characteristics	No.	%	No.	%	%
U.S. TOTAL	4,000	100.0	11,150	100.0	100.0
Census Areas					
Northeast	916	22.9	2,618	23.5	23.0
North Central	1,159	29.0	3,317	29.7	26.6
South	1,195	29.9	3,305	29.6	32.0
West	730	18.3	1,910	17.1	18.4
Census Regions–9 Way					
New England (NE)	205	5.1	587	5.3	5.6
Mid-Atlantic (NE)	711	17.8	2,031	18.2	17.4
East North Central (NC)	798	20.0	2,308	20.7	18.7
West North Central (NC)	361	9.0	1,009	9.0	7.9
South Atlantic (S)	609	15.2	1,679	15.1	15.9
East South Atlantic (S)	236	5.9	642	5.8	6.2
West South Atlantic (S)	350	8.8	984	8.8	9.9
Mountain (W)	188	4.7	495	4.4	4.6
Pacific (W)	542	13.6	1,415	12.7	13.8
Metro Area Size–8 Way					
Farm	165	4.1	466	4.2	3.9
Under 2,500	487	12.2	1,391	12.5	11.4
2,500–49,999	460	11.5	1,270	11.4	10.0
50,000–249,999	323	8.1	897	8.0	8.1
250,000–499,999	428	10.7	1,231	11.0	11.0
500,000–999,999	466	11.7	1,268	11.4	12.7
1–2 Mill.	561	14.0	1,508	13.5	13.7
2 Mill. & over	1,110	27.8	3,119	28.0	28.3
Household Income—6 Way					
Under $5,000	610	15.3	1,026	9.2	17.8
$5,000–$8,999	729	18.2	1,644	14.7	17.4
$9,000–$12,999	750	18.8	2,120	19.0	17.1
$13,000–$16,999	661	16.5	2,196	19.7	15.1
$17,000–$22,999	652	16.3	2,153	19.3	16.5
$23,000 & over	598	15.0	2,011	18.0	16.1
Education—Hh. Head—3 Way					
Grammar (under 9 yr)	609	15.2	1,409	12.6	20.6
High (9–12 yr)	1,861	46.5	5,299	47.5	48.3
College (over 12 yr)	1,530	38.3	4,442	39.8	31.1

TABLE 1 *Continued*

	Households and Household Members Distributed by Demographic Characteristics				
	Households in Sample		Persons in Sample		U.S. Census Households
Household Characteristics	No.	%	No.	%	%
Occupation—Hh. Head—4 Way					
White collar	1,455	36.4	4,505	40.4	32.5
Blue collar	1,219	30.5	4,098	36.8	33.1
Farmer	79	2.0	254	2.3	2.2
Not a worker	1,247	31.2	2,293	20.6	32.2
Homemaker Employment—2 Way					
Employed (6 mo or more)	1,445	36.1	3,928	35.2	NA
Not employed (less than 6 mo)	2,555	63.9	7,222	64.8	NA
Household Size—4 Way					
1 Person	791	19.8	791	7.1	20.6
2 Persons	1,317	32.9	2,634	23.6	30.6
3–4 Persons	1,359	34.0	4,771	42.8	32.9
5 or more	533	13.3	2,954	26.5	15.9
Presence of Children—6 Way					
None	2,345	58.6	4,263	38.2	57.8
Under 6 yr only	505	12.6	1,819	16.3	12.3
6–12 yr only	277	6.9	1,047	9.4	6.5
13–17 yr only	317	7.9	1,215	10.9	8.7
6–12 & 13–17 yr	232	5.8	1,196	10.7	6.7
Under 6 & other age-groups	324	8.1	1,610	14.4	8.0
Age of Homemaker—6 Way					
Under 25 yr	223	5.6	655	5.9	11.3
25–34 yr	886	22.2	3,167	28.4	22.4
35–44 yr	569	14.2	2,373	21.3	16.7
45–54 yr	635	15.9	1,970	17.7	17.3
55–64 yr	757	18.9	1,534	13.8	14.9
65 yr & over	930	23.3	1,451	13.0	17.4
Race—2 Way					
White	3,653	91.3	10,091	90.5	88.4
Nonwhite	347	8.7	1,059	9.5	11.6
Seasonal Totals					
Jul.–Sept. 1977	1,000	25.0	2,776	24.9	—
Oct.–Dec. 1977	1,000	25.0	2,718	24.4	—
Jan.–Mar. 1978	1,000	25.0	2,921	26.2	—
Apr.–Jun. 1978	1,000	25.0	2,735	24.5	—

TABLE 1 *Continued*

	Households and Household Members Distributed by Demographic Characteristics				
	Households in Sample		Persons in Sample		U.S. Census Households
Household Characteristics	No.	%	No.	%	%
Individuals by Age and Sex:					
Male—Total	3,142	78.6	5,127	46.0	48.6
Under 2 yr	169	4.2	171	1.5	1.5
2–5 yr	408	10.2	447	4.0	2.9
6–12 yr	501	12.5	603	5.4	5.8
13–17 yr	382	9.6	471	4.2	4.9
18–24 yr	380	9.5	426	3.8	6.6[a]
25–34 yr	791	19.8	797	7.1	7.5
35–44 yr	561	14.0	561	5.0	5.3
45–54 yr	528	13.2	529	4.7	5.2
55–64 yr	523	13.1	523	4.7	4.5
65 yr & over	595	14.9	599	5.4	4.4
Female—Total	3,950	98.8	6,023	54.0	51.4
Under 2 yr	159	4.0	160	1.4	1.4
2–5 yr	375	9.4	426	3.8	2.8
6–12 yr	493	12.3	606	5.4	5.6
13–17 yr	350	8.8	428	3.8	4.7
18–24 yr	436	10.9	466	4.2	6.6[a]
25–34 yr	917	22.9	919	8.2	7.7
35–44 yr	571	14.3	572	5.1	5.5
45–54 yr	645	16.1	648	5.8	5.6
55–64 yr	758	19.0	763	6.8	5.1
65 yr & over	1,002	25.1	1,035	9.3	6.4

NOTE: The U.S. Census Population Estimates are based on residents of the United States (includes institutional population).

[a] Includes all residents, whereas the Menu Census is based on household members only (excludes institutional population).

away from home for 14 consecutive days in daily diaries. Households are distributed uniformly throughout the year, with about 11 households starting on each day of the year. Thus, there are about 153 households reporting on each day of the year. Each quarter contains exactly 1,000 households. The sample is balanced within each quarter, as closely as possible, to the U.S. Census by various demographic characteristics, including region, household size, household income, and the like.

Households are invited to cooperate about 1 month before they will be needed, at which time they receive a yellow completed sample diary and a trial blank diary. When cooperators complete a trial diary, they are informed of any errors they may have made in reporting. When started, they are sent all 14 daily diaries and are instructed to begin reporting on a specified date. Incoming diaries are checked as received for accuracy and completeness, and write-backs are sent to the households to elicit additional details about the food used, or the nature of such use, as needed.

Following the fourteenth day, the household receives a diet questionnaire, in which it reports information about each individual member of the household, concerning weight, specific diets, foods encouraged to eat and encouraged to avoid, and the consumption of vitamin supplements. In addition, the homemaker receives a questionnaire dealing with attitude, awareness, and interest in various subjects related to food preparation and usage and to life-style.

The households are compensated with points for returning each diary or other form and for completing the entire study. These points tie in to their continuing compensation as members of NCP and therefore leverages on this other compensation that the household receives.

Transcription, Editing, and Processing

All information reported by the households in the daily diary and in the other questionnaires is coded, edited, and reported on a quarterly and on an annual basis. All foods are classified into about 65 major food categories and into as many as 99 different specific food items within each major category. Each item is further classified by three additional ways, depending on the specific major category. These additional classifications may refer to the presence of a particular additive, coating, flavoring, etc., or to the particular type of dish or way of serving, or to the specific form or source of the food as received by the household.

In addition, the package type in which the food came is classified, as well as the method of cooking or preparation, and the appliance used in preparation. Not only do we code every end dish as eaten, but also every ingredient used in its preparation.

All transcribed information is machine-edited against the code structure, to ensure the validity of codes assigned to particular products and to ensure that all ingredients of a particular dish are properly connected to that dish. In addition, checks are made to ensure that every household member is accounted for in each main meal of every day. For example, if a person is recorded as having eaten a meal away from home, a check is made to verify that some food is reported as eaten by that person away from home. The resulting transcribed records on tape form a complete image of the information reported by the household for each meal for every day. Thus, any analysis that could be specified on the basis of information written by the household in the diary could be carried out from the tape file.

Reports

Reports are produced at the end of each quarter and are delivered to subscribers about 4 months following the report period. Annual reports are processed and delivered immediately following the fourth quarter reports. Most subscribers follow up receipt of quarterly and annual reports with custom studies performed on various parts of the data base. These custom studies are usually executed with 2 to 6 weeks of authorization. They frequently involve the production of reports similar to the seven base reports, but executed on smaller or more finely defined subgroups of foods, or on special target households. These target households may be defined by the incidence of their usage of some foods in a particular way. For example, a study may be performed on the demographic classifications of households using both bottled soft drinks as well as powdered mixes in a 2-week period. Alternately, a study may be carried out, say, on the kind of starches served along with roast beef during the evening meal. As described above, special studies are also carried out on the cumulative exposure of individuals to specific additives or to particular nutrients from all foods eaten. Special analyses are carried out for many years following the execution of any one study and frequently involve developing trends in the pattern of use of a particular food product over 10 or 15 years.

Validity, Completeness, Accuracy, and Biases in the Data

It is relatively difficult to check the validity of Menu Census data for any particular product, because of the lack of easily obtainable independent reference information of similar detail. On the whole, based on 20 years of use by a large number of food processors and marketers, the Menu Census has proved to be a reliable reflection of patterns and trends in food preparation and usage.

As a rough check, some clients have estimated the coverage of specific product categories in the Menu Census as follows. An estimated average amount per eating occasion was multiplied by the frequency of eating of a specific product as reported in the Menu Census, and the resulting projected pounds of consumption in a 2-week period was compared to independently obtained average amount sold in an average 2-week period in that year. Such comparisons usually indicated a reasonable coverage of sales by the projected Menu Census data. However, it is known that certain product categories are not well reported in the Menu Census. These include products with a high frequency of consumption outside the direct knowledge of the homemaker or the reporter, such as snack foods, candy, alcoholic beverages, and the like. Similarly, consumption of candy and other snacks instead of regular school lunches by children away from home may not be properly reported to the homemaker. Forgetfulness may also affect reporting, especially of foods eaten by other household members away from home.

The quality of reporting in the Menu Census is significantly enhanced by the fact that all members are drawn from the National Consumer Panel and are required to have participated in that panel for over 6 months whenever possible. Thus, reporting of food preparation and consumption is done by "experienced reporters," who have learned how to enter information in diaries in specified columns and sections, and to identify foods, packages, brands, etc., using "standard" terminology rapidly and accurately.

Of course, as noted above, NCP households tend to be more interested in food purchasing, in economy, in "housekeeping," etc. Nevertheless, it seems unlikely that such characteristics would carry through in any appreciable degree to affecting adversely patterns of food preparation and eating. It seems likely that these biases may contribute at most to second- or third-order effects in information that is of significant use in the Menu Census.

Correlation Between Food Purchase and Usage by Menu Census Households

The Menu Census diary does not request the reporting of quantities used on any serving or eating occasion. Therefore, average amount per eating occasion must be obtained from other sources when Menu Census data is used to quantify amounts of food additives or other substances consumed through the food by individuals of various age-groups. The current method uses averages computed from the USDA 1965 Survey of Consumption by Individuals. We will shortly be able to use the data that has been collected by USDA on food intake by individuals in 1977–78.

Another method for quantifying the average amount per eating occasion may be available by correlating the average quantities of specific foods purchased by Menu Census households, as reported by them in the weekly NCP diaries in the same time periods during which they also reported food usage in the Menu Census daily diaries. For example, during the Fourth Menu Census, households reported their purchases of cottage cheese every week and also reported all usage occasions of cottage cheese during a 2-week period in the daily diaries. These two separate sources of information could be correlated, using a standard regression analysis model, for all 4,000 households, and thereby derive average estimated amounts per eating occasion for persons classified into several different age-groups. Since cottage cheese is a frequently purchased product, it appears that such estimates would be reasonably stable.

A project is currently under way to develop such estimates for a large number of food categories whose purchases were reported in NCP during the period from July 1972 through June 1973, overlapping the Fourth Menu Census period. No results are as yet available from this study. If this study results in reliable estimates of consumption, then a good link would have been established between purchase information and consumption information for the same household. Therefore, one could track food consumption information indirectly by estimating it from purchase data. Since purchase data is usually less expensive to collect, one could collect Menu Census information only periodically, and in between one could follow up with observations of purchases of selected key products, from which estimates would be derived of the consumption of these same products by individuals in various age-groups.

In addition, since the relation between food purchases by households and movements of foods earlier in the pipeline is already well understood, one could use higher levels of aggregation of food movement at these earlier points in the distribution system to monitor emerging changes in food consumption. This possible relationship between aggregate and detail information has previously been discussed in the first workshop of this committee.

Collecting Data on American Food Consumption Patterns: An Anthropological Perspective

CLAIRE MONOD CASSIDY

According to Samuel Beck, English propaganda that the French lived on frogs and salad were implicity believed. Nathaniel Tracy, to entertain properly the admiral and officers of the French fleet, had the swamps of Cambridge searched for green frogs, which were served whole in the soup at a formal dinner. The first officer who struck one with his spoon fished it out, held it up, and exclaimed: ''Mon Dieu! une grenouille!'' The fascinated company embarrassed Tracy by roaring with laughter.

R. O. Cummings,
The American and His Food, 1940:30.

INTRODUCTION

The purpose of this paper is to consider how the anthropological perspective can contribute to the development of superior methods for collecting data on U.S. (''American'') food consumption patterns. I will review selected literature related to (1) anthropological studies of food habits among U.S. Americans and (2) theoretical orientations and techniques employed by anthropologists that are of utility in the assessment of consumption patterns in urbanized society.

ANTHROPOLOGY IN NUTRITION

The anthropologist is fundamentally interested in *variability* (its sources in the social, cultural, historical, and biological spheres) and *change* (its patterning, constancy, rate alterations). These subjects are approached classically using variants of the cross-cultural comparative method. Though anthropologists formerly concentrated their research in prehistoric and "exotic" or non-Western societies, contemporary interest increasingly focusses on urban and urbanizing peoples worldwide. Sociocultural anthropology developed and refined the now widely used nonquantitative technique of *participant observation* for eliciting information on behavior, beliefs and expectations from respondents.

Montgomery (1978:43) summarizes orientations to research he finds shared by anthropologists. His five points are worth quoting at length:

> 1) The recognition of the necessity to understand people in their own terms; 2) The maintenance of a healthy suspicion that what people say or believe bears no necessary relationship to what they do; 3) The recognition that much of "culture" or "cultural behavior" is expressed in non-verbal ways; 4) The recognition that some of "culture" or "cultural behavior" is "unconscious" in that its existence, performance, or patterning is manifested without the actor's conscious or express awareness; 5) The recognition that, in any group of people, significant variations among and within individuals with respect to both beliefs and actions are to be expected.

Cancian (1977) lists characteristics of anthropological science that make it especially effective in gleaning or disseminating information to/from non-Western peoples. (Here I shall use "non-Western" not as a geographic term but as one distinguishing philosophical positions *not* characterized by faith in and dependence upon "science" and "rationalism," hence potentially present among Americans.) Anthropologists are, then, scientists who are interested in discovering exceptions, in gaining width of perspective (holism) and in practicing patiently paced research strategies. They are often antiestablishment (or, at least, skeptical of the reality of "universal" truths).

Anthropologists have long been interested in foods, ways of using foods ("foodways," "food habits"), and nutrition. Earlier studies (e.g., Richards 1932, 1939; DuBois 1944; Honigmann 1961; Firth 1966; Rappaport 1968) considered foods as part of a larger ethnological picture and provided good data on attitudes and dietary content but typically little quantitative data adequate for assessing nutritional status. The latter subject has become of greater concern recently, especially with the emergence of the subdiscipline of nutritional anthropology.* Since numerous able reviews of this subject and

*Nutritional anthropology focusses primarily on questions of nutrition and emphasizes the biocultural ecology approach. Students of the *anthropology of food* use the semiotic and folkloric approaches and are interested primarily in habits and beliefs associated with food use. The Committee on Nutritional Anthropology was founded in 1974. It is a branch of the Society for Medical Anthropology, recognized by the American Anthropological Association. Its newsletter is the *CommuNicAtor*. Within the International Union of Nutritional Scientists (IUNS) is the International Committee on Nutritional Anthropology (ICNA), while within the its history have recently appeared, I will not review it further here (Wilson, 1973; Netting, 1974; Arnott, 1976; Fitzgerald, 1976; Freedman, 1977; Johnston, 1977; Haas and Harrison, 1977; Montgomery, 1978; Montgomery and Bennett, 1978; Wilson, 1978).

Anthropologists interested in foods and nutrition have used several theoretical orientations, including the *historical* (e.g., Cummings, 1940; Simoons, 1967; Chang, 1977); *folkloric* (analysis of material culture associated with food preparation, use, and storage); *humanitarian* (expressed as a concern with world hunger, which leads to consideration of food habits primarily as they affect the probability of malnutrition); *biocultural; ecology;* and *semiotics*. The biocultural ecology approach requires that foods and food habits be analyzed with respect to their capacity to promote adaptation to the natural environment. The functional interpretation argues that under normal circumstances human groups will tend to find and practice food habits that optimize food distribution and maximize food value. An important implication of this approach is that the apparently "irrational" food habit may, when interpreted with greater care, prove rational. Take, for example, the refusal of milk ("nature's most nearly perfect food"!) by many malnourished peoples. This act appeared irrational until the genetic distribution of adult lactase insufficiency was discovered (McCraken, 1971). The hot–cold dichotomy, a health and nutrition patterning system probably descendant from Greek ideas of humoral pathology and still important in many areas of the world, is currently believed to have no basis in physiological fact. But Lindenbaum (1977) mentions in passing emerging data that contradicts this interpretation. In the semiotic approach, "Food has been studied not for itself, but as a medium for social and for cognitive expression . . . " (Singer 1978:3).

Singer (1978) defines three research goals for nutrition in anthropology, including in ascending inclusive order: (1) to use semiotic insights—"the various treatments of food as symbol"—to understand "eating . . . as an expressive act which . . . is trying to say something about something"; (2) to study "how the cultural system fits with the food production and nutritional systems"; and (3) to analyze the historical transformations of food systems. "Internal dialectic, external pressure, and the necessities of survival may combine to lead to a changing fit between cultural, productive, and

---

International Union of Anthropological and Ethnological Scientists (ICAES) is the Commission on the Anthropology of Foods (ICAF) and the Committee on the Anthropology of Foods. Montgomery and Bennett (1978) list two journals and four newsletters devoted to the subjects of food, nutrition, and anthropology; more recent appearances include *Appetite, The Journal for Research on Intake, Its Control and Its Consequences* (international); *The Digest, a Newsletter for the Interdisciplinary Study of Food* (Graduate Group in Folklore and Folklife, University of Pennsylvania); and *Foodtalk* (San Francisco).

biological spheres thus creating new ways of eating and of feeding" (1978:3–4). These ideas are significant to the analysis of U.S. food consumption patterns because they suggest both how broad must be our approach to collection and how potentially useful the final product may be *if* we can isolate and identify the more significant sources of pressure for change (or stability) and use these for prediction or intervention.

FACTORS ASSOCIATED WITH FOOD CONSUMPTION

What Is A Food?

A food is at once a substance that provides energy or nutrients to maintain body function, a substance capable of assuaging hunger pangs, and a substance defined as "edible." These meanings are not necessarily equally recognized by users, and in practice the third meaning is usually the most significant to the largest number of people.

Edibility itself is not a simple concept, a fact recognized by the Committee on Food Habits of the National Research Council (1945), which said:

> . . . [from the class of all] edible materials [some] are classified as inedible, edible by animals, edible by human beings, but not my kind of human being, edible by human beings such as self, and finally edible by self. These classifications are further reinforced by various sorts of attitudes—that materials which are not eaten are defiling, wicked to eat, coarsening, would alter one's status, etc.

The list in the second part of this section suggests the large number of factors that (potentially) affect the actual consumption of food in the family and by individuals.

The terms "food habits" and "foodways" are sometimes distinguished (Cussler and DeGive, 1952), but recently have been used interchangeably as "habits of a group that reflect the way a culture standardizes behavior of the individual in the group in relation to food, so that the group comes to have a common pattern of eating" (Lowenberg *et al.*, 1974:117).

Leininger (1969) attempts to distinguish *food universals,* valid cross-culturally from nonuniversals. Leininger's nine food universals are characteristics of food use presumed to be present and functioning in all human groups. Food is: (1) "used to provide body energy and statisfy biophysiological hunger"; (2) used to initiate and maintain interpersonal relationships with friends, kinsmen, and strangers; (3) a determinant of the "nature and extent of interpersonal distance between people;" (4) used to express social and religious ideas; (5) used to "illustrate social status, prestige, group achievements"; (6) used to help individuals cope with psychological stresses and needs; (7) used to reward, punish, or otherwise influence the behavior of others; (8) used to "influence the political and economic status of a group"; and (9) used to "detect, treat and prevent social, physical and cultural behavior deviations and illness manifestations" (Leininger, 1969:*passim*).

The nonuniversals, in contrast, assort food use by (1) culture-associated preferences (affected by various taboos, symbols, social structure, environmental availability, etc.); (2) relationship to the supernatural, magic, sorcery, and curing (or health maintenance); (3) social stratification; (4) appearance and manner of serving; (5) the "internal metabolic environment and its interaction with the external environment" (Leininger, 1969:*passim*).

When we ask what is used as food by lay people, we find the list includes some items formally considered nonnutritive, such as edible earths, laundry starch, ice cubes, caffeinated beverages, hard liquor, coca leaf or betel nut, tobacco, and so forth (cf., Wilson, 1978). Wison considers these worth including in any survey of food habits because some may add important amount of nutrients (e.g., calcium from the typical betel nut preparation), while others may interfere with good nutritional status (e.g., cigarettes, coca.).

Choice and Availability of Food in the Family

The actual choice of food made by families and individuals is governed by many factors, some of which are listed in Table 1. The list is garnered, in part, from earlier attempts to assess what information must necessarily be collected to wholly understand food consumption patterns, American or other (cf., Eggan and Pijcan, 1943; Manual for the Study of Food Habits, 1945; Mead, 1964; Leininger, 1969; Christakis, 1963; Jerome, 1969a; Pangborn, 1975; Haas and Harrison, 1977; Wilson, 1978). The fact that these factors appear as a list does not mean they do not interact with each other; in fact, they overlap and share feedback relationships, the details of which remain to be fully worked out.

METHODS

A number of attempts have been made to detail methodologies appropriate to the collection of food consumption data (The Problem of Changing Food Habits, 1943; Manual for the Study of Food Habits, 1945; Mead, 1955; Christakis, 1973), while several authors have made suggestions of information that might be included in such methodologies (e.g., Eggan and Pijcan, 1943; Mead, 1949, 1964; Lee, 1957; Pangborn, 1975; Jerome, 1969a,b; Haas and Harrison, 1977; Montgomery, 1978; Wilson, 1978; cf., Table 1).

TABLE 1 Factors Affecting Food Choice and Availability

Category	Item	Comment
Biologic	Genetics of food choice	Populations differ genetically in ways significant to food choice, e.g., lactase deficiency and adult milk use (Bunce, 1969; Davis, 1969; McCracken, 1971); PTC tasting and cabbage family attractiveness (Fischer, 1967)
	Limits of human adaptability	Age, sex, altitude, temperature, body size and composition; significance of agriculture as a recent alteration in food source and type (cf., Stini, 1971; Haas and Harrison, 1977)
Ecologic	Soil fertility, water micronutrient content, ecozone variety, climate	Seasonal variation in the food supply
Economic	Production, transportation, & distribution	Politics of food supply; societal stability; fossil fuel availability
	Family income	Storage facilities
Sociologic	Classifications	Ethnicity; religion; class; caste; sex; age; occupation; education; rural–urban
	Rate of change in society	Local homogeneity of culture; isolation; access to advertising and nutrition information; access to alternate food sources
Household familial	Acquisition decisions	Purchasing power; technical ability to acquire (shopping habits, gardening, hunting, gathering knowledge); technical ability to prepare (status kitchen, food preparer education); family structure
	Distribution decisions	Daily work schedule; sex, age, and health of members; food-sharing behavior; idiocultures
Cognitive	Conceptualizations of edibility and food categorizations	Sacred, ordinary, and "fun" foods; sexuality enhancing foods; health-promoting foods; health-damaging foods; allowable combinations of foods; folk classifications of foods; color and shape associations.[a]
	Body image	Preference for "fat" or "lean" shapes by age, sex; demonstrations of social status by body habitus (Cassidy, in press)

[a] In the United States (and elsewhere), "white" chicken meat has higher status value than "dark," white rice than brown, white bread than dark (though we are possibly witnessing a change in status for some of these). Mead (1949) tells how shape of the serving dish may take precedence over its contents, hence nonmeat combinations will be accepted as meal "main dishes" if they are served in the appropriate container.

American society is vast, complex (i.e., multiple interacting networks of production, distribution, education, control, and accession), heterogeneous, mobile, individualized. We face a large problem when we decide to develop a methodology that will distill from this mass a utilitarian (i.e., usable for purposes of prediction) description of American food consumption patterns

Anthropologists have classicaly concentrated their research in small and non-Western societies. There were two good reasons for this. A small society is "graspable"—researchers can feel some confidance that the whole (at least most) of its character

Anthropologists have classically concentrated their research in small and non-Western societies. There were two good reasons for this. A small society is "graspable"—researchers can feel some confidence that the whole (at least most) of its character can be discovered and perhaps described and understood; its boundaries are defined, hence so is the necessary extent of the anthropological inquiry. Second, the non-Western society is (usually) different enough from their own society to force the researchers to take little for granted, to rediscover, and to question their own categories of the "normal," "ordinary," and "natural."

The two advantages of working in the small and the distant are missing when we choose to analyze our own society. Therefore, in developing a methodology, we must pay particular attention to (1) *identifying biases* (cultural, educational, paradigmatic) that affect our ability to recognize significant data and to design effective research strategies and (2) deciding *how much data* we want to collect.

Identifying Biases

The failure to recognize biases can cause incomplete data collection or the development of hypotheses based on invalid assumptions. In either case, the predictive value of findings is significantly reduced. For example, in Belize, Lowland Maya feast periodically on a pig's head. Men, the butchers and for these occasions the cooks, serve themselves the muscle portions, while women receive the fat, eyes, and brain. During my fieldwork there, I was told by another anthropologist that this distribution pattern was "another example of males overpowering females"—here, specifically of taking the nutritionally better portions for themselves. This interpretation reflects bias and is probably proportionately invalid. The biases include the American one against organ foods and fat but towards protein (especially muscle) foods, and an ethnological one, which, expressed as an assumption, reads "men hold most of the power worldwide." This latter has the evidence of many earlier ethnographic works behind it and appears to have been "proven" by recent research that shows women of child-bearing age frequently receive disproportionately unbalanced diets (cf., Rosenberg, 1973). Yet it has not, in my opinion, received adequate scrutiny. In any case, because of the unrecognized presence of these biases, this researcher reached premature closure on an ethnological problem. Alternate interpretations include phrasing the male–female power relationship in a form accessible to research, such as, "Where is the locus of women's power?"; and recognizing the important nutritional components of fat, eyes, and brain (fatty acids, fat-soluble vitamins), which are, in fact, relatively scarce in the typical daily Lowland Mayan diet. In this way we are led to see that the food distribution *favors women nutritionally,* and at the same time *symbolically reifies* an important masculine–feminine distinction, that of strength (meat is a "strong" food in Belize). Finally, because fat is *highly desirable* in most nonindustrialized societies (and among subgroups in our own society), the provision of fat to women cannot imply any male lack of regard for women.

Other assumptions—or tendencies of mind—that are common and necessary to avoid in developing methodology are the very subtle ones of:

- considering the norms of one's own group as normal (i.e., confusing norm and normal), which easily leads to viewing variability as *ab*normality or, in nutritional terms, as *inadequacy;*
- considering the group with which we identify (e.g., white middle class, nutrition professionals) as homogeneous with regard to food consumption patterns; or
- accepting as real the existence of reference persons, modal personalities, culture types, and so forth.

For both of the latter it is important to recognize that the amount of *intra*cultural diversity is frequently greater than the amount of intercultural diversity (Pelto and Pelto, 1975), especially as the detailed examination of groups inevitably leads to heightened sensitivity to subtleties of preference and use.

Arensberg and Niehoff (1975) distinguish characteristics of American culture that are particularly important as they affect food use or our ability to design research. Though racially, ethnically, religiously, and occupationally heterogeneous, Americans express a rather narrow range of opinion on moral, political, economic, and social subjects. They are quite conforming with regard to language, hygiene, dress, diet, basic skills, land use, community settlement, and recreation, facts Arensberg and Niehoff associate with our efficient mass education system. Status differences are present, but not very marked, and fall mainly along lines of occupation, education, and financial worth. There is considerable geographic and occupational mobility. The family is commonly nuclear, with few children. In spirit the country is strongly secular and rationalistic, and displays strong interest in comfort (often expressed in terms of cleanliness), achievement, and success. The latter may be had by effort and efficient use of time (i.e., speed, precision). Anyone can succeed (egalitarianism); personal liberties exist and should not be infringed upon (individualism). Humans are almost infinitely perfectible; the person should attempt to improve himself. Progress not only may be had, but is almost a constant; the future orientation is also expressed in the accent on youthfulness and in an overwhelming concern with providing for children. Humanitarianism—or concern for the welfare of others—is highly valued, but is usually expressed impersonally. Twofold judgements (work: play, moral:immoral, civilized:primitive, practical:impractical, adequate: inadequate) are characteristic—this puts the world of values into absolutes and tends to force users into positions of exclusiveness.

"Science" is a belief system and method that has been, in the last 100 years, so acceptable to Americans as to have become almost a faith. It is based in rationalism, and profits from American emphases on speed, accuracy, and the future orientation. What is labelled "scientific" is also almost inevitably labelled "progressive." However, the twofold judgement is replaced in science by the concept of continua, an emphasis on gradual variation, and often by a desire to avoid judgement except in flexible (rejectable) terms.

Contrasts to modal American and nonmodal American and non-Western systems may be found in Arensberg and Niehoff (1975), Jelliffe and Jelliffe (1976), and Cancian (1977).

Jerome (1969a) distinguishes seven "themes" in American culture (individualism, democracy, capitalism, industrialism, pluralism, youthfulness, leisure) and shows how these affect food habits. For example, individualism and the emphasis on self-expression are shown through autonomy in food selection and consumption and the use of "image" foods that symbolize reward, reassurance, nostalgia, power, strength, etc. To ask Americans to give up certain foods for therapeutic or preventive purposes is to ask them to forsake independence and autonomy, even the democratic process; dependency is much feared by Americans. Capitalism stimulates demand through advertising; competition builds available variety of foodstuffs. Pluralism means that certain foods and food habits are at the core of the diet and are recognized as "American" by outsiders (e.g., hamburgers, sliced white bread, fruit drinks, carbonated beverages, apples, milk), while others (secondary food habits) reflect the basic eating patterns of subcultures (regional, ethnic, religious) or the incorporation of nontraditional food items or whole cuisines into total foodways (accessory eating patterns). The interest in leisure is played out through the increasing use of restaurants and snack foods. Youthfulness is emphasized by the avoidance of fat and "fattening foods" and the use of low-calorie or "health" foods.

Much work on American food habits, though able to provide guidance, is nevertheless rather impressionistic (e.g., Mead, 1943; Joffe, 1943; Lee, 1957; Mitchell *et al.*, 1968; Lowenberg, 1974). However, some details on local groups has been provided through the important and interesting work of Lewin, 1943; Bennett *et al.*, 1942; Jerome, 1969b, 1975.

Defining Research Boundaries

Food consumption analysis can be carried out at several levels of increasing precision, including the national, regional, community, neighborhood, household, and individual (the "idioculture" of food habits). The job of this workshop is to detail methods to collect information on the household and the individual, hence our research boundaries are already partially specified. Nevertheless, we must decide (1) how to conceptualize and categorize the enormous amount of information available on households and individuals and (2) how to discover what potential information we will consider irrelevant to our purpose, for research on cultural subjects is almost infinitely extendable.

There are at least four reasons for collecting data on American food consumption habits:

- to learn more about American culture;
- to assess the nutritional adequacy of diets and status of the population;
- to identify the malnourished (presumably to intervene); and
- to introduce "new" foods or recipes or alter proportions to dietary items for economic or public health reasons.

A weighting of the importance of these four (which I do not wish to imply by this list) would provide a first step toward identifying research boundaries.

Included as problems here are the needs for:

- a measure of homogeneity in food use; this could be approached through the use of the core, secondary core, etc., categorizations as quantified by Jerome (1975);
- some built-in characteristic(s) to ensure flexibility so that change may be identified and described.

Some Minor Points

Included here are some ideas that simply do not fit handily elsewhere.

Sexist or racist terminology must be avoided in designing research instruments. For example, Christakis' (1963) dietary methodology section distinguishes between "homemakers" who are female and "heads of household'' who are male and on question forms does not provide for working women (a majority of American women) or one-parent families. The decision to classify families on the basis of male occupation alone can be severely biasing. In the same source, all infants and children are referred to as ''he'' while their caretakers are called ''she.''

New categories to include ''health,'' ''natural,'' and ''ethnic'' foods and use of ''food supplements'' (e.g., yeast, ''Tiger's milk,'' vitamins, etc.) need to be developed.

Instruments such as ''Basic 7'' or ''Basic 4'' charts should contain in each category a broad enough range of foods to include those familiar to people of all ethnicities. The categories should be defined in nutritional terms, not in terms of cultural ideals.

Research instruments, where possible, should be precoded for the computer. Computer programs can be developed early to handle the data; some sophisticated ones that permit mapping (e.g., of subtleties of food use countrywide) are now fairly readily available. It is important to reach predecisions on the handling of subjective data before mass surveys begin.

Techniques Used by Anthropologists

Included in this section are a small number of papers by anthropologists or nutritionists with anthropological training that describe novel, or employ adaptations of classical, techniques and that provide insights of utility to our present purpose. Wilson (1978) points out that the approaches used by anthropologists are considerably individualized and suggests that there has been little attempt at standardization because so few such studies have been done thus far.

The classical anthropological technique is *participant observation*. This technique requires the researcher to live with and participate in the lifestyles of study populations. The potentials for discovering subtleties and for detailing the systematics of cultural behavior are excellent, particularly in small and well-bounded populations such as those having band or tribe organization, or among people identified by community or caste membership. The technique requires highly trained personnel and the devotion of large blocks of time (months, years) to research. It becomes progressively less manageable as population size or sociopolitical complexity rise. It does not typically provide quantified data. These characteristics are technical liabilities in urbanized societies where information on large groups is wanted quickly and cheaply. However, a number of adaptations of participant observation have been developed over the years that overcome many of these problems.

These adaptations involve, first, selecting a specific problem-topic on which to focus research. Techniques from other disciplines are sometimes added to the research plan to guide interviews or to provide quantified data. Thus: (1) Respondents may be followed and observed with regard to the problem-topic intensively for brief periods without the use of interviews. Wilson (1974) recommends this approach as superior for collecting dietary data on toddlers who cannot respond well to a recall technique. A possible drawback, especially in a mobile society, is that if the child is taken elsewhere the researcher may not be able to follow. (2) Questionnaire-guided topical interviews may be combined with brief periods of socializing with respondents (e.g., Jelliffe *et al.,* 1962). (3) Living near respondents and making frequent visits may be combined with depth interviews and/or the use of questionnaires on the problem-topic (e.g., Bennett *et al.,* 1942; Jerome, 1969b, 1975). (4) Living with respondents may be combined with use of depth interviews on the problem-topic and the collection of quantified data (e.g., McArthur, 1962; Cassidy and Stavrakis fieldwork, 1973–74).

In each of these variations, researchers select population subgroups from whom to elicit details on the problem-topic. Selection occurs on many bases, from the decision to use a small number of "key informants" who are willing (self-selection) and able (time and language are common barriers) to spend extended periods in contact with the researcher to random samples of special-interest groups (e.g., female heads-of-household) who then further self-select according to willingness to be interviewed or to permit the anthropologist to observe them in their homes.

Interviews may be partially or wholly structured; anthropologists typically prefer the "open-ended" style, because it gives more leeway for the inclusion of respondent opinion and belief and decreases the risk of missing significant information, because of unrecognized biases introduced by the questionnaire-maker.

Bennett *et al.* (1942) completed a now-classic study of a southern Illinois rural community in which they used partially structured interviews and free-association techniques to elicit information on food habits. Late in their study, they employed paired-comparison to cross-check accuracy of knowledge derived from interview. They spent 3 months on the project, visited all over the study area, but lived with only one of the subgroups they identified ("lower hills" people). They introduced the concepts of *core* (staple, regularly used foods), *secondary core* (recently introduced store-bought foods), and *peripheral* (very recent additions stimulated by special economic conditions) diets as means to order the mass of descriptive data they collected. The result was excellent, but possibly limited in two ways: There was no measure of nutritional adequacy of diets; the choice to live with one group produced better understanding of that group and possibly altered relationships with other and rival groups in the area.

Jerome (1969b, 1975) studied how the food habits and conceptualizations of food altered for rural black Americans as they migrated north to major urban centers and how black Americans in a mid-Western urban center adapt their diets to supermarket variety and personal food preference. Both studies employed multiple visits to respondent households and partially structured depth interviews, and both required several months of research time with subsequent computer work-up. Jerome borrows Bennett *et al.*'s terminology but alters and quantifies their definitions. Thus *core* includes the essentials of the diet, "consumed 2–3 times per day by ⩾25% of respondent households"; *secondary core* includes the food "consumed about once a week by ⩾25% of respondent households"; *peripheral* includes the foods "consumed 1–2 times per month by ⩾25% of households"; and *ceremonial/marginal* includes "foods and beverages on the borderline of either being completely excluded from the diet or only included on very few occasions by ⩾75% of respondent households" (Jerome, 1975:92–93). This study approach combines several characteristics that make it possibly of greatest utility for the collection of food consumption data on Americans.

McArthur, to quote Wilson (1978:142), "combined participant observation and detailed budgetary studies to several households during one period with "dropping in" at meal preparation times to see what was to be served and on occasion to share a meal with that family." The resultant data was semiquantified.

Cassidy and Stavrakis, working with Lowland Maya in Belize, lived 12 weeks (1973–74) in one village, ate regularly in one household, participated fully in accessible village activities, made a census of households, and interviewed all female heads of household in multiple-depth interviews that covered the topics of obstetrical and health history, child health histories, food habits and beliefs, agricultural production, and sources of other food. We then selected eight households for a quantified dietary survey and, using a team of trained undergraduate aides, collected recipes and weighed food and plate waste for *all* family members in each of the selected households for two 24-hour days. The work included following children to observe snacking behavior and using recall to elicit snacking behavior and the content of meals away from home from adults. Nutritional status was estimated from Guatemalan food tables prepared by INCAP. This approach provided quite complete information on the food beliefs and habits of a whole village and on the food intake of approximately 1/4 of the village.

The participant observation aspect of this research worked well, but the in-home weighing was not wholly successful. This was mainly because, though we took precautions to minimize our impact and to minimize dietary change coincident with our visits, we knew our presence was disturbing, hence food use on survey days altered (mostly by protein enrichment). An adjustment of the weighing portion of the approach would make it less obtrusive yet provide equally (if not more) useful data. In the households selected for intensive study, a week's food use could be collected by arriving unannounced (having previously obtained permission) to observe and weigh, let us say, three morning meals, four noon meals, and three evening meals in a week, collecting at the same time recall information on the nonobserved meals for that day. Snacking behavior could be collected by recall, or by some combination of recall and following. Collection and analysis of resultant data requires use of the computer. Such an approach would be useful where very detailed and precise information was wanted, especially to establish "normality" guidelines, or to answer questions about, e.g., family food distribution patterns (sex, age, preference), the nutritional adequacy of different diets, or the amount of variation in the diet. The technique should be equally applicable to analysis of any well-defined population group.

Another route to knowledge of food use is through the analysis of household refuse. Adapting their method and theory from archaeology, the Garbage Project of Tucson, Ariz. (Harrison *et al.*, 1975; Rathje and Harrison, 1978) has shown that food waste behavior varies by socioeconomic status and ethnicity and can serve as a measure of responsiveness to business cycles. The method has several advantages. It is a "nonreactive measure of behavior"—that is, it measures "what people did, not what they think they did" (Harrison *et al.*, 1975:13). It is inexpensive and demands no time or cooperation from subjects. It permits household food waste to be estimated quantitatively. However, it provides no information on food beliefs or family food distribution patterns.

Chassy *et al.* (1967) used the Guttman Scale of increasingly less inclusive steps to weight the importance of various foods in the diet and the change in weighting with urbanization in a model industrial town in Mexico. This scale can also be used to measure the effect of contact with different cuisines. The technique has been used by Sanjur *et al.* (1970) to assess child-feeding practices in a Mexican village, and DeWalt and Pelto (1977) modified it to consider nutritional adequacy indirectly by assessing the degree of complexity of the diet, also in rural Mexico. This approach requires the use of a structured questionnaire on food consumption. It produces information on dietary patterning but no quantified data. However, it requires no highly trained intereviewers and permits information on large numbers of subjects to be collected.

Table 2 summarizes these techniques (necessarily somewhat subjectively) according to criteria deemed important to the development of methodology by the Food and Nutrition Board's Committee on Food Consumption Patterns (letter of July 24, 1978).

TABLE 2 Preliminary Assessment of Utility of Some Food Consumption Collection Techniques

Techniques[a]	1	2	3	4	5	6
Sample size handled	large	moderate	large	small	moderate	moderate
Individuals emphasized?	no	no	no	yes	potentially	yes
Reaches specific populations	yes	yes	yes	yes	yes	yes
Identifies those at risk	moderate	moderate	low	high	high	high
Ease of collection	high	high	high	moderate	moderate	moderate
Flexibility of collection	low[c]	low[c]	uncertain	low	high	high
Quantified data?	no	no	yes	yes	yes	yes
Categorical data?	yes	yes	yes	yes	yes	yes
Subjective data?	no	some	no	yes	yes	yes
Personnel[b]	–	–	–	+/–	+	+
Reliability	moderate[d]	moderate[d]	high[d]	high	high	high
Predictive value	moderate	moderate	high[d]	moderate[e]	high	high
Rapid handling ease	high	high	high	moderate[f]	moderate[f]	moderate[f]
Cost-effectiveness	moderate	moderate	high	moderate	fairly high	fairly high

[a] Technique 1 = Structured Questionnaires and Guttman Scale; 2 = Structured Questionnaires and Socializing; 3 = Household Refuse; 4 = Person Following; 5 = Depth Interviews and Food Use Observation or Quantification; 6 = Participant Observation and Food Use Quantification.
[b] A "+" indicates highly trained personnel are necessary for some part of the research (usually the unstructured interviews); a "–" indicates that personnel trained only briefly can administer questionnaires or make observations.
[c] Flexibility is considered low where structured questionnaires are used.
[d] High or moderate for households or groups, not for individuals.
[e] Predictive value is dependent on sample size and other items.
[f] Subjective data requires transformation to objective categories, hence computerization may get complex.

A Possible Approach to the Collection of Food Consumption Data

Table 3 summarizes, in a very preliminary manner, an approach to the collection of food consumption data on the American population. It is anthropological (specifically ethnological) in outlook as it emphasizes participant observation and the collection of "subjective" data. It is suggested as a platform for discussion.

SUMMARY

Because American society is large, heterogeneous, and mobile, we set ourselves a peculiarly difficult problem in deciding to design a methodology for

TABLE 3 One Possible Approach to Collection of Food Consumption Data on Americans, a Tabulation Intended for Discussion

Sequence of Data Collection	Step I	Step II	Step III
Main assumption(s)	"We know nothing of the food consumption patterns (of group x)."[a]	"Subjective data can be adequately coded into categories."	"The major potential sources of bias in the study have been identified and adjusted for." "All the questions we consider important have been provided for."
Goal(s)	collect as much data as possible	identify and specify desired and necessary data; develop instruments to get data faster and cheaper; test adequacy of instruments to assess accuracy[b]	collect as much specific data as possible

Sample size coverable	small	medium	large
Time required proportionate to usuable data collected	moderate	moderate	small
Subtlety of data collected	high	falling	low[c]
Personnel training	advanced	moderate	moderate
Main techniques	some variety of participant observation, open-ended interviews; detailed measurement of food use and waste	semi-structured interviews with long single or multiple visits; simpler assessment food use and waste	apply instruments developed in steps I and II

[a]This assumption helps avoid the use of possibly outdated information.

[b]Test adequacy of instruments on *same* populations (but different persons) as Step I to assess accuracy of instruments.

[c] But if research instruments were well designed, it is still high, and specifically, high enough for the intended purpose.

the collection of food consumption data. The anthropological perspective is valuable as it emphasizes the existence and importance of intracultural diversity, the constancy of change, the special characters of the Americans and the American scientist that must be adjusted for in research design, and a small number of techniques, mostly nonquantitative, that provide irreplaceable detail on subjective aspects of culture.

REFERENCES

Arensberg, C. M., and A. N. Niehoff. 1975. American cultural values. Pages 363–378 *in* The Nacirema, readings in American culture. Little Brown Co., Boston.

Arnott, M. L. 1975. Gastronomy, the anthropology of food and food habits. Mouton, The Hague.

Bennett, J. W., H. L. Smith, and H. Passin. 1942. Food and culture in southern Illinois, a preliminary report. Am. Soc. Rev. 7:645–660.

Bunce, G. G. 1969. Milk and blindness in Brazil. Nat. Hist. 78:52–53.

Cancian, F. 1977. Can anthropology help agricultural development? Culture Agric. 1(2):1–8.

Cassidy, C. M. In press. The clinical significance of imaging body fat as beautiful. Soc. Sci. Med.

Chang, K., ed. 1977. Food in Chinese culture: Anthropological and historical perspectives. Yale University Press, New Haven.

Chassy, J. P., A. G. van Veen, and F. W. Young. 1967. The application of social science research methods to the study of food habits and food consumption in an industrializing area. Am J. Clin. Nutr. 20:56–64.

Christakis, G., ed. 1963. Nutritional assessment in health programs. Am J. Public Health 63(Suppl.), November 1963.

Cummings, R. O. 1940. The American and his food. University of Chicago Press, Chicago.

Cussler, M., and M. L. DeGive. 1952. Twixt the cup and the lip. Twayne Publications, Inc., New York.

Davis, A. E., and T. D. Bolin. 1969. Milk intolerance in Southeast Asia. Nat. Hist. 78:53–55.

DeWalt, D. M., and G. H. Pelto. 1977. Food use and household ecology in a Mexican community. *In* T. K. Fitzgerald, ed. Nutrition and anthropology in action. Van Gorcum, Assen, The Netherlands.

DuBois, C. 1944. The people of Alcor, a social–psychological study of an East Indian island. University of Minnesota Press, Minneapolis.

Eggan, F., and M. Pijcan. 1943. Some problems in the study of food and nutrition. Am. Indigena 3:9–22.

Firth, R. 1966. Housekeeping among Malay peasants, 2d ed. Athlone Press, London.

Fischer, R. 1967. Genetics and gustatory chemoreception in man and other primates. Pages 61–81 *in* M. R. Kare and O. Maller, eds. The chemical senses and nutrition. Johns Hopkins University Press, Baltimore.

Fitzgerald, T. K., ed. 1977. Nutrition and anthropology in action. Van Gorcum, Assen, The Netherlands.

Freedman, R. L. 1977. Nutritional anthropology: An overview. *In* T. K. Fitzgerald, ed. Nutrition and anthropology in action. Van Gorcum, Assen, The Netherlands.

Haas, J. D., and G. G. Harrison. 1977. Nutritional anthropology and biological adaptation. Ann. Rev. Anthropol. 6:69–182.

Harrison, G. G., W. L. Rathje, and W. W. Hughes. 1975. Food waste behavior in an urban population. J. Nutr. Educ. 7:13–16.

Honigmann, J. J. 1961. Foodways in a Muskey community: An anthropological report on the Attawapiskat Indians. Department of Northern Affairs and Natural Resources, Ottawa, Canada.

Jelliffe, D. B., J. J. Bennett, R. H. R. White, T. R. Cullinan, and E. F. P. Jelliffe. 1962. The children of the Lugbara, a study in the technique of paediatric field surveys in tropical Africa. Trop. Geogr. Med. 14:33–50.

Jerome, N. W. 1969a. American culture and food habits, communication through food in the U.S.A. *In* J. Dupont, ed. Dimensions of nutrition. Colorado Associated University Press, Boulder.

Jerome, N. W. 1969b. Northern urbanization and food consumption patterns of Southern-born Negroes. Am. J. Clin. Nutr. 22:1667–1669.

Jerome, N. W. 1975. Flavor preference and food patterns of selected U.S. and Caribbean blacks. Food Technol. 29(6):46–51.

Joffe, N. 1943. Food habits of selected sub-cultures. U.S. Bull. Natl. Res. Counc. No. 108.

Johnston, F. W., ed. 1977. Anthropological aspects of human nutrition. School of American Research, Santa Fe.

Lee, D. 1957. Cultural factors in dietary choice. Am. J. Clin. Nutr. 5:166–170.

Leininger, M. 1969. Some cross-cultural universal and non-universal functions, beliefs, and practices of food. *In* J. Dupont, ed. Dimensions of nutrition. Colorado Associated University Press, Boulder.

Lewin, K. 1943. Forces behind food habits and methods of change. Pages 35–65 *in* Natl. Acad. Sci./Natl. Res. Counc. Bull. No. 108. Washington, D.C.

Lindenbaum, S. 1977. The "Last course": Nutrition and anthropology in Asia. Pages 141–155 *in* T. K. Fitzgerald, ed. Nutrition and anthropology in action. Van Gorcum, Assen, The Netherlands.

Lowenberg, M. E., E. N. Todhunter, E. D. Wilson, J. R. Savage, and J. L. Lubawski. 1974. Food and man, 2d. ed. John Wiley & Sons, New York.

McArthur, A. M. 1962. Malaya 12. Assignment report, June 1958–Nov. 1959. World Health Organization, Regional Office for the Western Pacific, Manila, The Philippines.

McCracken, R. D. 1971. Lactase deficiency: An example of dietary evolution. Curr. Anthropol. 12:479–517.

Manual for the study of food habits. 1945. Natl. Acad. Sci./Natl. Res. Counc. Bull. No. 111. Washington, D.C.

Mead, M. 1943. The problem of changing food habits. Pages 20–34 *in* Natl. Acad. Sci./Natl. Res. Counc. Bull. No. 108

Mead, M. 1949. Cultural patterning of nutrition related behavior. J. Am. Diet. Assoc. 25:677–680.

Mead, M., ed. 1955. Cultural patterns and technical change. Mentor, New York.

Mead, M. 1964. Food habits research: Problems of the 1960's. Natl. Acad. Sci./Natl.Res. Counc. Bull. No. 1255. Washington, D.C.

Mitchell, H. S., H. J. Rynbergen, L. Anderson, and M. V. Dibble, eds. 1968. Cooper's nutrition in health and disease, 15th ed. J. B. Lippincott, Philadelphia, pp. 144–154.

Montgomery, E. 1978. Anthropological contributions to the study of food-related cultural variability. Pages 42–56 *in* S. Margen and R. A. Ogar, eds. Progress in human nutrition, Vol. II. Avi Publishing Co., Inc., Westport, Conn.

Montgomery, E., and J. W. Bennett. 1978. Anthropological studies of food and nutrition: The 1940's and the 1970's. *In* W. Goldschmidt, ed. The uses of anthropology. American Anthropological Association Special Publication No. 11.

Netting, R. M. 1974. Agrarian ecology. Ann. Rev. Anthropol. 3:21–56.

Pangborn, R. M. 1975. Cross-cultural aspects of flavor preference. Food Technol. 29(6):34–36.

Pelto, P. J., and G. H. Pelto. 1975. Intracultural diversity: Some theoretical issues. Am. Ethnol. 2:1–19.

The problem of changing food habits. 1943. Committee on Food Habits, Natl. Acad. Sci./Natl. Res. Counc. Bull. No. 108. Washington, D.C. 177 pp.

Rappaport, R. A. 1968. Pigs for the ancestors, ritual in the ecology of a New Guinea people. Yale University Press, New Haven.

Rathje, W. L., and G. G. Harrison. 1978. Monitoring trends in food utilization: Applications of an archaeological method. Fed. Proc. 37:49–54.

Richards, A. I. 1932. Hunger and work in a savage tribe, a functional study of nutrition among the southern Bantu. G. Routledge and Sons, London.

Richards, A. I. 1939. Land, labour and diet in northern Rhodesia: An economic study of the Bema tribe. Oxford University Press, London.

Rosenberg, E. 1973. Ecological effects of sex-differential nutrition. Unpublished oral presentation to American Anthropological Association, New Orleans.

Sanjur, D., J. Craviota, and A. G. van Veen. 1970. Infant nutrition and socio-cultural influence in a village in central Mexico. Trop. Geogr. Med. 20:443–451.

Simoons, F. J. 1967. Eat not this flesh, food avoidances in the Old World. University of Wisconsin Press, Madison.

Singer, E. A. 1978. Guest editorial: Thoughts on the new foodways. *In* The Digest, a newsletter for the interdisciplinary study of food 1(2):2–4.

Stini, W. A. 1971. Evolutionary implications of changing nutritional patterns in human populations. Am. Anthropol. 73:1018–1030.

Wilson, C. S. 1973. Food habits: A selected annotated bibliography. J. Nutr. Educ. 5(Suppl. 1)(1):38–72.

Wilson, C. S. 1974. Child following: A technic for learning of food and nutrient intakes. J. Trop. Pediat. Environ. Child Health 20:9–14.

Wilson, C. S. 1977. Research methods in nutritional anthropology: Approaches and techniques. Pages 62–68 *in* T. K. Fitzgerald, ed. Nutrition and anthropology in action. Van Gorcum, Assen, The Netherlands.

Wilson, C. S. 1978. Developing methods for studying diet ethnographically. Pages 141–148 *in* E. E. Bauwens, ed. The anthropology of health. C. V. Mosby Co., St. Louis.

Individual Variation in Intake of Nutrients by Day, Month, and Season and Relation to Meal Patterns: Implications for Dietary Survey Methodology

HAROLD B. HOUSER *and* HELEN T. BEBB

Common methods for collection of dietary intake of individuals include the food record or diary kept by the individual or a close family member. This method has been used by us extensively in a variety of settings including yearlong studies of food intake (Houser *et al.*, 1969; Witschi *et al.*, 1970a,b; Bebb *et al.*, 1971; and Bebb *et al.*, 1972). Our goal in these latter studies has been to establish for each individual a group of data that would be representative of a subject's usual or average or "typical" diet. Our observations indicate the marked variation of an individual's intake over time, as well as the variation between individuals. Because of this variation, it becomes difficult to assess the frequency and duration of data collection needed for a representative picture of an individual's usual or average food intake.

The dietary intake of 127 adults who kept 3-consecutive-days diary records of their food intake at 12 intervals for a year are examined in this paper from the standpoints of individual variability and the numbers and frequency of records that are representative of the year's intake. In addition, from the data we will evaluate the ability to predict intake by selected food items, the relation of food-intake history to recorded intake, and the utility of modal patterns of intake.

SUBJECTS

Study Group I consisted of 32 men and 41 women who were chronically ill with multiple sclerosis and living at home. The subjects represented various stages of the disease from mild to severe. Ages ranged from 29 to 62 years; mean age for women was 43 years; mean for men, 44 years.

Study Group II consisted of 54 healthy males who were employed in executive or management positions in a single corporation. They ranged in age from 23 to 62 years; mean age, 44 years.

Study Group III consisted of 28 males, all professionals and executives, who were participating in a physical fitness program. They ranged in age from 27 to 58, with a mean age of 45.1 years.

METHODS

General Data Collection

A diary record was kept by each subject for a period of 3 consecutive days at approximately monthly intervals (Houser *et al.*, 1969). For Group I, the recording days were selected to ensure a sample of weekdays, weekend days, and holidays throughout the year. For Groups II and III, recording days were selected at random.

All foods and beverages were recorded by the subjects in common measures, i.e., cups or number of items by count. Special attention was given to notation of brand names, or unusual ingredients. Date, day of the week, and time and place of the meal or snack were recorded.

The diary method demands a great deal of cooperation and motivation from subjects, particularly with 36 days of recording. Subjects in Group 1 showed 33 out of 106 subjects who did not complete records for 1 year or who had records considered unsuitable—illness (3), death (1), withdrawal from study (4), and moving (1) accounted for 9 subjects. Ten did not submit satisfactory records and 14 did not return or complete records on schedule. Group II had a much higher success rate. Of 55 subjects who began the study, only 1 withdrew and the remaining 54 completed satisfactory records. One Group II subject submitted only 11 records (33 days). Six Group III subjects withdrew (Table 1).

Of those who finished, the mean number of days to return records to nutritionist remained consistent over the year. For all groups the average number of days ranged from 3 to 4 for all sets of records. Subjects were called, if necessary, about returning records or if specific food items on the record need clarification. The fact that 94 out of 127 subjects received from 0 to 3 phone calls over the entire year also helps establish the records as reliable and helps demonstrate the feasibility of the study method.

When records were processed for computer analysis, each food or beverage item consumed was filed so that it could be identified by subject number, the day of record, date of record, day of the week, item number for the day, meal period code, actual time of intake, food table identity number used for nutrient calculations, usage code, which explained, for example, if the margarine was used as a spread or used over a vegetable, and a code for

TABLE 1 Number of Subjects in Dietary Intake Studies with Diary Recording for 1 Year (161 Subjects) or 6 Months (36 Subjects) by Completion of Record Status

		Subjects			
	MS	Executives	Fitness	Total	
Failure to Complete	No.	No.	No.	No.	%
Unsatisfactory records	10	0	0	10	5.0
Nonadherence to schedule	14	0	5	19	9.0
Subject withdrew	9	1	3	13	7.0
Successful completion	73	54	28	155	79.0
TOTAL	106	55	36	197	100.0

quantity and type of measure. This complete identification of our food items permitted flexibility in computer calculation of results.

For each subject, daily nutrient intake was averaged for the 36-day study period. Calories and grams of protein and fat from animal and plant sources, of carbohydrate from refined sugar and from natural sources, and alcohol were calculated, as were average daily amounts of calcium, phosphorus, iron, vitamin A activity from beta-carotene and preformed A, thiamin, riboflavin, niacin, and ascorbic acid.

METHODS USED TO EVALUATE METHODOLOGY AND VARIATION

To Examine Variation Over Time

Difference in means For each subject, the 36 days of daily intake were reviewed 5 different ways, using Student's t-test to show difference in means. T-values were evaluated for significance at the 0.05 and 0.01 levels. In addition to the nutrients listed above, total protein, total fat, and total carbohydrate were calculated and tested as well, giving a total of 21 variables tested for each subject. If a significant difference in means was found, both the level of significance and the direction of the difference were noted.

Test No. 1: To evaluate a possible effect of differences in eating during summer and winter, study days falling during May through October were averaged and compared to the average of study days occurring during November through April.

Test No. 2: To evaluate whether we could have collected data for 3 days a month at intervals of every other month instead of every month, we numbered each 3-day set from 1 to 12, and tested the means of sets numbered 1, 3, 5, 7, 9, and 11 (odd numbered sets) with the means from the 3-day sets numbered 2, 4, 6, 8, 10, and 12 (even numbered sets).

Test No. 3: To evaluate whether subjects eat differently on weekdays than they do on weekends, the average for all weekdays (Monday through Friday) was compared to the average for all weekend days (Saturday and Sunday).

Test No. 4: To evaluate the possibility of collecting only 1 day a month instead of 3 days a month for a period of 1 year, we compared the mean obtained from all first days of each 3-day set with the mean from the remaining second and third days of each 3-day set.

Analysis of Variance Analysis of variance was used to measure individual reporting consistency over the twelve 3-day sets. Variation within the 3-day set was compared to the variation among the sets. Only 19 of the above 21 variables were tested. Alcohol calories were included with calories from other carbohydrate, and total vitamin A activity was omitted.

To Examine Variation in Meal Patterns

Number of meals and snacks reported per day were totaled and the mode assigned to the meal pattern observed most often for each individual. Other calculations included amount and percent of calories consumed during meals and snacks.

Methods to Develop Multiple Regression Equations to Predict Dietary Intake

In order to form our food groups for the equations all items in our food table (HVH-CWRU Nutrient Data Base), approximately 1,600, were considered as possible predictors. Because the computer program for determining the regression equations considered a maximum of 79 independent variables at a time, it was necessary to either eliminate items or group them on the basis of nutrient composition.

First, single food items were combined into 495 "specific item categories." Combinations were made on the basis of similar composition; for example, several forms of canned pineapple, i.e., slices, chunks, tidbits, and crushed, were all grouped as canned pineapple and three sizes of whole oranges were grouped as "fresh whole oranges." Then, a frequency count was made of these food categories consumed by the group of multiple sclerosis men and women to determine: (1) the number of subjects reporting the 495 categories and (2) the number of days each category was reported. Two hundred forty-one categories (about 700 single food items) were eliminated on the basis that less than 10 percent of the group reported the category at least once during the 36 days. Additional elimination of 94 groups was accomplished following the criteria of: (1) an item must have been consumed by about 30 percent of the subjects over the 36 days or (2) if fewer than 30 percent, then the item had to have been reported on more than 50 occasions over the 2,628 days observed. Five exceptions were later made to include the specific item categories of lamb chops, haddock, pike, salmon, and wheat thins to give a more complete representation to the lamb, fish–shellfish, and cracker groups.

The final single food item count was 510 and these made up 160 specific item categories. A final count of the 510 single items showed that 92 percent of the total food items reported by the Group I subjects were included in the 510 items. A comparison with Group II showed these items accounted for 90 percent of reported items. To further facilitate calculations, another grouping was made to condense the 160 categories into 69 food groups.

All items in the food table are in common household measure, and this is how subjects were requested to report quantities of food consumed. For most items in the food table, it is possible for subjects to report quantitities in more than one type of measure, including (1) weight, (2) volume by measure from a teaspoon to a quart, or (3) by count (where appropriate) of the item itself, e.g., three pineapple rings, four brussel sprouts, two medium pork chops trimmed of fat, or two scoops of ice cream. Each of the 69 food groups was assigned a basic quantity unit and for each subject, amounts of each of the 510 items in the 69 groups were converted from the subject's reported quantity to a fraction of the basic quantity unit. For each subject, an average daily intake for each food group was calculated.

METHODOLOGY FOR REGRESSION EQUATIONS

The dependent variables included the average daily intakes of calories, animal protein, plant protein, animal fat, plant fat, refined carbohydrate, other carbohydrate, and alcohol. Input data from the 113 men (32 Group I men, 54 Group II men, and 28 Group III men) were used, so that any differences in intake between men and women would not bias the results.

To arrive at the final regression equation, the following procedures were followed for each dependent variable:

1. Initial determination of the number of independent variables necessary in each regression formula (N): Through stepwise regression analysis, 15 variables out of the 71 were entered into the equation, F-level for inclusion, 0.01; F-level for deletion, 0.001. The variables were listed in the order as they entered the equation together with the multiple correlation coefficient (R) and the multiple R-square (RSQ); variable number 1 explaining the greatest amount of variance. Then starting with variable number 1, the number of variables was increased by one until: (a) the RSQ reached 70 or greater (ideally 75 or greater); (b) the increase in RSQ showed a reasonable

break point; and, (c) at this time, for reasons of later computational restrictions, the total number of variables did not exceed 8.

2. Selection of the best variables to be considered for each equation: Stepwise regression may or may not select the best combination of variables to predict the dependent variable, or there may be another set which would give nearly the same R and RSQ, which would be just as acceptable. In order to test this, for each dependent variable, up to 15 independent variables were selected using these criteria: (a) when the number of independent variables for each equation (N) was determined, all variables from the first through the Nth were automatically included as 1 of the possible 15 total to be selected; (b) the simple correlation between each dependent variable with all independent variables was calculated. Additional variables were selected on the basis of a relatively high correlation with the dependent variable (approximately $R = >0.315$); and (c) reasonableness of obtaining intake data about the variable from the subject.

3. Determination of all possible combinations (up to N variables at a time) of the 15 independent variables, and calculation of the residual mean square (RMSQ). Variables were taken one at a time, two at a time, etc. until N number of variables at a time was reached.

4. Combinations of variables having the lowest RMSQ were compared with stepwise regression results and the best combinations of variables were selected for each dependent variable.

Methods for Collecting Diet History

At the end of the study year, the 73 subjects in Group I completed a dietary history through a structured interview with the study dietitian. The history was directed toward the frequency of consumption of specific food items on a usual basis such as never, once a week, or daily (Table 2). For some items quantity was also obtained. For each frequency code, 95 percent confidence limits of a Poisson distribution were calculated based on 36 sample days and the actual frequency determined from the 36 days of diary recording were tested against the probability assigned to the frequency code.

Fifty-one specific foods were analyzed in this manner and the observed frequency was determined to be less than, the same as, or more than the response indicated by history.

Meal Patterns

Food intake on the diary recording forms was recorded by the subject as taken at meals or between meals. We accepted the subject's recorded state-

TABLE 2 Subject Choices for Response to Questions About Usual Frequency of Consumption of Specific Foods

Code	Frequency
0	never
1	once a month or less
2	2–3 times a month
3	once a week
4	2–4 times per week
5	5–7 times per week
6	once a day
7	2–3 times a day
8	4–6 times a day
9	>6 times a day

ment even though recorded intake at a snack might exceed that at a preceding or following meal.

The meal and snack periods were coded using seven code numbers:

Code Number	Indicates Food Eaten:
1	Before breakfast
2	Breakfast
3	Between breakfast and lunch snack
4	Lunch
5	Between lunch and dinner snack
6	Dinner
7	After dinner snack

If food was consumed at several different times between meals, only one between meal snack was coded.

RELIABILITY AND VALIDITY OF DATA

Subjective assessment (by the study dietitian) of the recorded data and of the subjects' reliability, the compliance with schedules and instructions, and the reasonableness of the analyses of intake as previously reported (Witschi *et al.*, 1970; Bebb *et al.*, 1972) have led us to accept the diary records as representative of each individual's usual intake during the recording period. The relationship between the intake of the 73 subjects with multiple sclerosis and the fatty acid composition of their subcutaneous fat has also been examined and lends support to the validity of the data (Table 3).

TABLE 3 Rank Order Correlations (r_s) of Total Diet-Iodine-Index (Range 50.5–86.1) with Serum Cholesterol and Adipose Tissue Fatty Acid Proportions

	Cholesterol	Palmitic	Oleic	Linoleic
Males (32)	−0.07	−0.19	−0.08	+0.57[a]
Females (41)	+0.14	−0.12	−0.18	+0.33[b]
All subjects (73)	+0.07	−0.21	−0.11	+0.53[c]

[a] 1 P <0.05.
[b] 2 P <0.005.
[c] 3 p <0.0005.

Representative sampling of weekdays and weekend days is suggested by the data in Figure 1, which show that the proportion of weekend days in each subject's daily records falls within a 95 percent confidence interval for the true proportion of weekend days.

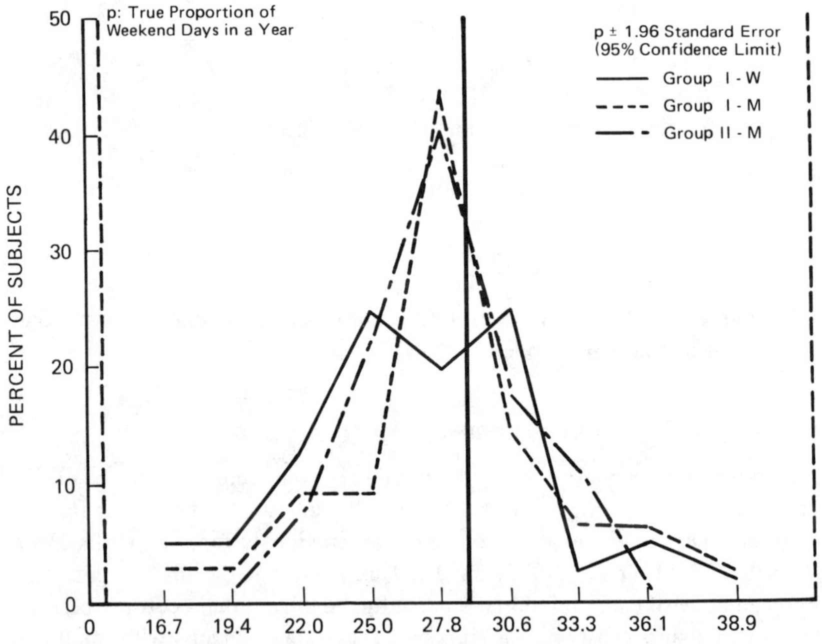

FIGURE 1 The distribution of subjects by the percent of weekend days in the 36 days of diary recording.

RESULTS

The number of multiple sclerosis and executive subjects showing significant variation by analysis of variance among their 12 sets of records for each of 18 nutrients and calories is shown in Table 4. While the relative rank of nutrients varied between two groups, Spearman's rank order correlation coefficient is significant; on the strength of this the two groups are combined to show the percent of individuals showing significant variation for each of the nutrients. Table 5 shows the distribution of subjects by the number of items per subject showing significant differences among the 12 sets. The median number of items for the groups is three.

The significant differences in mean values for 20 nutrients and calories by the several comparisons are shown in Table 6. The direction of the differences, that is a significant increase or decrease, is also shown in this table. The least number of differences occurred when the first recording days of each set were compared to the second and third days combined. Odd sets compared to even sets, May–October compared to November–April, the

TABLE 4 Significant Variation Among 12 Sets of 3-Day Records for Individual Nutrients in 127 Adults

	Significant Differences			
	MS[a]	Executive[a]	Total	
Nutrient	No.	No.	No.	%
Vitamin A	8	7	15	11.8
Riboflavin	8	7	15	11.8
Niacin	9	5	14	11.0
Animal protein	10	4	14	11.0
Total protein	12	4	16	12.6
Animal fat	14	10	24	18.9
Carotene	14	2	16	12.6
Iron	15	8	23	18.1
Thiamin	16	7	23	18.1
Phosphorus	20	10	30	23.6
Total fat	20	8	28	22.0
Plant protein	21	12	33	26.0
Plant fat	23	12	35	27.6
Carbohydrate, refined	24	6	30	23.6
Ascorbic acid	24	11	35	27.6
Total carbohydrate	25	15	40	31.5
Calcium	25	12	37	29.1
Carbohydrate, natural	26	12	38	29.9
Calories	29	11	40	31.5

[a]Rank order: $r_s = 0.74$ P <0.01.

TABLE 5 Number of Subjects with Significant Variation in 19 Nutrients Among 12 Sets of 3-Day Food Diaries

Number of Items Varying per Subject	Subjects MS No.	MS Cum. %	Executive No.	Executive Cum. %	Total No.	Total Cum. %
≥0	8	11	8	15	16	13
1	6	19	11	35	17	26
2	7	29	9	52	16	39
3	10	42	7	65	17	52
4	8	53	4	72	12	61
5	12	70	7	85	19	76
6	7	79	1	87	8	83
7	4	85	2	91	6	87
8	3	89	3	96	6	92
9	1	90	1	98	2	94
≥10	7	100	1	100	8	100
TOTALS	73		54		127	

first 6 months of records compared to the last 6 months,* and weekdays compared to weekends, respectively, showed increasing numbers of differences. The individual nutrients, with the exception of carotene and ascorbic acid, followed patterns similar to the overall patterns. The cumulative percent of subjects by the number of items showing significant differences is shown in Figure 2. Sixty-four percent of the subjects had no nutrients with significant differences between the first and second and third days of records and 80 percent had one or less difference; all subjects, except one, had four or less significant differences. The other curves show increasingly higher percentages of subjects with larger numbers of differences in the same direction as shown in Table 6.

A comparison between the analysis of variance results and the differences in means testing is shown in Table 7. By the goodness of fit chi square test, the patterns in each of the three groups for day one versus days two and three and for weekday versus weekend days show no significant differences.

The food items used in the final multiple regression equations are shown in Table 8. Fifteen of the 25 variables entered into more than one equation; COOKIE appears in five of the equations for the eight dependent variables. The number of variables could have been one less for several equations by our original criteria but the necessary presence of the variable in another equation and a slight increase in the correlation coefficient, R, by its inclu-

*Most subjects completed their first set of records in late spring or early summer. Therefore there is considerable overlap of the seasonal and early and late records.

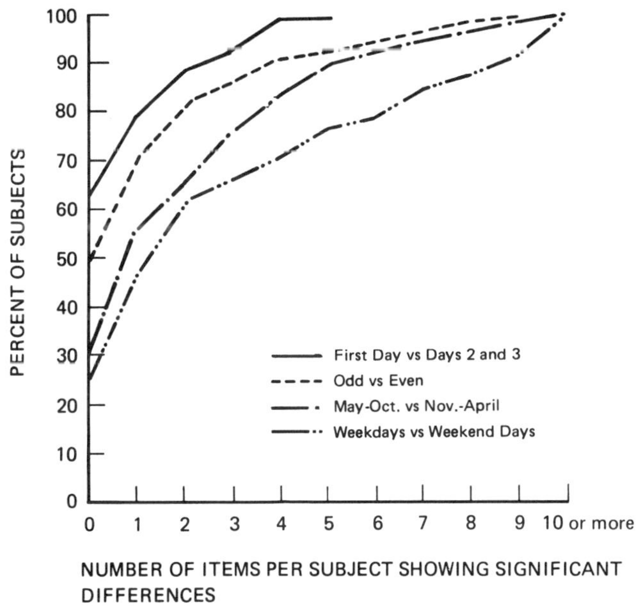

FIGURE 2 Cumulative percent of subjects by number of individual nutrients with significant difference in means in 12 sets of 3-day food diaries.

sion led us to include it in the equation. With the exception of one variable, animal and plant protein showed different sets of independent variables. This was also true for animal and plant fat and refined and other carbohydrate. For alcohol, food groups other than the three types of alcoholic beverages explained extremely small amounts of the variance so the total number of variables was limited to two.

For each of the 25 food variables in the equation, Table 9 shows the mean units of food consumed over 36 days. Some differences are apparent. The greatest consumption of beer and whiskey was shown by the executive group. There was a greater use of margarine and less butter by the executive men and the physical fitness group (a possible time trend, as the food consumption data for the general U.S. population showed a similar shift during the 1960's). Sandwiches were frequently reported as lunch items for the multiple sclerosis group and this explains the slightly higher group means for bread and the hot dog–lunchmeat category.

The multiple correlation coefficients (R) and the percent of variance accounted for by the equation (R^2) are presented in column one of Table 10. Multiple R's ranged from 0.89 to 0.99; the lowest R^2 was 0.79 (plant fat and

TABLE 6 Number of Subjects Showing Significant Difference for Five Analyses Using Student's T-Test

Test Variable	May–Oct. vs. Nov.–Apr.			First 6 Months vs. Last 6 Months			Odd Sets vs. Even Sets			Weekday vs. Weekend Days			1st Day vs. 2d & 3d Days		
	T[a]	I[b]	D[c]	T	I	D	T	I	D	T	I	D	T	I	D
Calories	17	7	10	18	7	11	12	4	8	29	26	3	4	2	2
Protein															
Total	14	4	10	19	8	11	8	2	6	24	18	6	9	2	7
Animal	16	5	11	19	8	11	7	3	4	24	19	5	7	1	6
Plant	16	9	7	20	9	11	11	3	8	18	14	4	5	2	3
Fat															
Total	15	8	7	20	7	13	7	4	3	30	29	1	7	3	4
Animal	13	4	9	12	3	9	10	5	5	26	25	1	5	0	5
Plant	10	7	3	10	5	5	9	4	5	18	13	5	6	3	3
Carbohyrdrate															
Total	21	11	10	13	9	4	17	7	10	19	16	3	5	2	3
Natural	19	10	9	21	10	11	13	3	10	19	12	7	5	2	3
Refined	15	7	8	18	7	11	7	6	1	21	16	5	3	1	2

Alcohol	8	2	6	9	4	5	3	2	1	23	20	3	1	0	1
Calcium	18	8	10	21	8	13	9	3	6	19	11	8	4	2	2
Phosphorus	17	7	10	23	9	14	12	3	9	22	16	6	6	1	5
Iron	13	9	4	24	11	13	9	4	5	22	17	5	8	2	6
Total Vitamin A	8	0	8	10	2	8	8	4	4	7	6	1	2	2	0
Preformed A	5	3	2	5	0	5	6	3	3	16	14	2	2	0	2
Beta-carotene	11	3	8	16	6	10	7	4	3	7	3	4	4	2	2
Thiamin	10	4	6	18	7	11	9	2	7	18	15	3	6	2	4
Riboflavin	14	5	9	20	6	14	8	5	3	20	17	3	6	3	3
Niacin	8	1	7	15	6	9	6	2	4	18	15	3	3	1	2
Ascorbic acid	16	6	10	16	8	8	4	3	1	7	3	4	1	0	1
SUBTOTALS															
Group IF	97	37	60	116	30	86	56	13	43	83	60	23	28	12	16
Group IM	91	52	39	105	51	54	44	20	24	98	82	16	21	10	11
Group IIM	96	31	65	136	59	77	82	43	39	226	183	43	50	11	39
TOTALS	284	120	164	357	140	217	182	76	106	407	325	82	99	33	66

[a] = Total.
[b] = Increased.
[c] = Decreased.

TABLE 7 Comparison of Results for Analysis of Variance with Results from Five Tests to Determine Variation Using Student's t-Test for Difference in Means

	By Analysis of Variance, No. of Subjects with 0 or 1 Items	Percent of Difference in t-Test	By Analysis of Variance, No. of Subjects with 2 or 3 Items	Percent of Difference in t-Test	By Analysis of Variance, No. of Subjects with 4 or more Items	Percent of Difference in t-Test
May Through October Versus November Through April						
Group I — F	12	14.4	10	17.5	19	68.1
Group I — M	3	7.7	13	37.4	16	54.9
Group II—M	24	34.4	15	25.0	15	40.6
First 6 Months Versus Last 6 Months						
Group I — F	12	15.5	10	4.3	19	80.2
Group I — M	3	4.8	13	36.2	16	59.0
Group II—M	24	25.0	15	38.2	15	36.8
Odd Sets Versus Even Sets						
Group I — F	12	12.5	10	21.4	19	66.1
Group I — M	3	0.0	13	25.0	16	75.0
Group II— M	24	34.1	15	39.0	15	26.9
Weekdays Versus Weekend Days						
Group I — F	12	33.7	10	20.5	19	45.8
Group I — M	3	14.3	13	45.9	16	39.8
Group II— M	24	41.6	15	33.2	15	25.2
Days 1 Versus Days 2 and 3						
Group I — F	12	42.9	10	21.4	19	35.7
Group I — M	3	19.0	13	38.1	16	42.9
Group II— M	24	46.0	15	36.0	15	18.0

TABLE 8 Independent Variables Used in One or More Regression Equations

Independent Variables	Abbreviations	Dependent Variables							
		Calories	Animal Protein	Plant Protein	Animal Fat	Plant Fat	Refined Carobohydrate	Other Carbohydrate	Alcohol
Bread and Cereals									
Bread	BREAD	Yes		Yes				Yes	
Buns—hot dog–hamburger	BUNHDH		Yes	Yes	Yes	Yes			
Cake	CAKE			Yes		Yes	Yes		
Cereal—dry	CERDRY							Yes	
Cookie	COOKIE	Yes		Yes		Yes	Yes	Yes	
Doughnut	DOUNUT	Yes				Yes			
Pie	PIE					Yes	Yes		
Fruits and Vegetables									
Potatoes	POTATO	Yes				Yes		Yes	
Vegetables—cooked	VEGCKD	Yes		Yes				Yes	
Meat									
Beef	BEEF		Yes		Yes				
Chicken	CHICKN	Yes	Yes						
Eggs	EGGS		Yes						
Fish—shellfish	FISHSH		Yes						
Hot dog—lunchmeat	HDLCHM		Yes		Yes				
Port—ham	PORKHM				Yes				
Dairy									
Butter	BUTTER				Yes				
Margarine	MARG					Yes			
Milk—whole	MKWB		Yes		Yes				
Other									
Beer	BEER	Yes		Yes				Yes	Yes
Coke	COKE						Yes		
French dressing—oil	FRDROL					Yes			
Maple syrup	MPLSYP							Yes	
Soup	SOUP			Yes				Yes	
Sugar	SUGAR						Yes		
Whiskey	WHISKEY	Yes							Yes

TABLE 9 Group Mean of Total Intake Over 36 Days for 25 Independent Variables

Independent Variable	Unit	Group Mean for Total Number of Units			
		MS Men	Executive Men	Physical Fitness Men	All Men
Bread and Cereal					
Bread	1 Slice	98.2	86.4	64.7	84.3
Buns—hot dog–hamburger	1 Bun	5.1	11.9	13.3	10.4
Cake	1 Piece	4.6	3.3	2.9	3.6
Cereal—dry	1 Cup	6.5	8.6	11.2	8.7
Cookie	1 Cookie	25.7	18.8	21.6	21.4
Doughnut	1 Roll/Doughnut	9.7	13.1	12.2	12.0
Pie	1 Piece	4.5	4.5	2.8	4.1
Fruits and Vegetables					
Potatoes	1 Cup	16.1	15.2	12.6	14.8
Vegetables—cooked	1 Cup	11.2	12.6	9.9	11.5
Meat					
Beef	1 Ounce	19.9	38.5	24.2	29.8
Chicken	1 Ounce	22.8	28.9	31.3	27.8
Eggs	1 Egg	25.1	24.9	19.2	23.5
Fish—shellfish	1 Ounce	19.9	18.2	24.6	20.1
Hot dog—lunchmeat	1 Ounce	45.6	35.5	35.1	38.2
Pork—ham	1 Ounce	24.2	24.9	15.1	22.3
Dairy					
Butter	1 Teaspoon	74.5	52.3	34.6	54.0
Margarine	1 Teaspoon	17.4	33.6	35.1	29.4
Milk—whole	1 Cup	25.4	16.0	10.2	17.1
Other					
Beer	1 12-Ounce Bottle	11.8	49.7	8.9	29.2
Coke	1 Cup	14.3	12.9	9.8	12.5
French dressing—oil	1 Tablespoon	10.6	19.1	30.2	19.6
Maple syrup	1 Tablespoon	4.3	7.6	5.2	6.1
Soup	1 Cup	8.2	9.8	9.6	9.3
Sugar	1 Teaspoon	94.0	77.2	25.6	69.0
Whiskey	1 Ounce	12.5	53.9	23.6	35.1

TABLE 10 Correlation Coefficient (R) and R^{2a} for Predicted Intake Versus Actual Intake for All 113 Men Plus Four Individual Groups Using Formula Developed for 113 Men to Predict Variable Values

	All Men (113)		MS Men (31)		Executive Men (54)		Physical Fitness Men (28)		MS Women (40)	
Variable	R	R^2	R	R^2	R	R^2	R	R^2	R	R^2
Calories	0.90	0.81	0.71	0.50	0.77	0.59	0.68	0.46	0.78	0.61
Protein										
Animal	0.90	0.81	0.82	0.67	0.80	0.64	0.43	0.18	0.69	0.48
Plant	0.91	0.83	0.81	0.66	0.81	0.66	0.62	0.38	0.81	0.66
Fat										
Animal	0.93	0.86	0.90	0.81	0.89	0.79	0.67	0.45	0.63	0.40
Plant	0.89	0.79	0.79	0.62	0.82	0.67	0.81	0.66	0.88	0.77
Carbohydrate										
Refined sucrose	0.94	0.88	0.84	0.71	0.87	0.76	0.77	0.59	0.68	0.46
Other	0.89	0.79	0.64	0.41	0.80	0.64	0.65	0.42	0.79	0.62
Alcohol	0.99	0.98	0.97	0.94	0.98	0.96	0.86	0.74	0.90	0.81

[a] R^2 is the percent of the total variance explained by the regression equation.

other carbohydrate). Multiple R's and R^2's are lower when the 113 men are divided into their respective study groups and the correlation coefficients were calculated for actual versus predicted intake in each separate group.

As a test, the data from the 40 women were used with the regression equations for the 113 men. Predicted intake was correlated with actual intake; multiple R's range from 0.63 to 0.90 for the eight dependent variables. Except for animal fat, all are higher than those for the physical fitness group, but for calories, plant protein, plant fat, and other carbohydrate, they compare well with the other two groups of men.

The regression equations for each of the eight variables are shown in Table 11.

In Table 12, the actual group means and the group mean of predicted values are shown with their standard deviations for the four study groups. With few exceptions, the group means from predicted values are either approximately equal to or less than means from actual values and standard deviations are generally of the same magnitude.

The modal patterns of meals and snacks and the number of subjects with each pattern are shown in Table 13. The most frequent modal pattern, three meals with three snacks, was present in 63 (50 percent) of our subjects. The distribution of all subjects by the percent of days each subject consumed food by his modal pattern is shown in Table 14. Only 40 percent of subjects had 50 percent or more of their days as modal pattern days and only 15 percent had three-fourths or more days at their modal pattern.

TABLE 11 Regression Equations Based on Dietary Intake for 113 Men

Dietary Factor	Regression Equations[a]
Calories	3.8 (BREAD) + 6.3 (BEER) + 16.2 (DOUNUT) + 25.5 (POTATO) + 7.7 (COOKIE) + 3.7 (WHISKEY) + 7.9 (CHICKN) + 14.1 (VEGCKD) + 513.4
Animal protein	0.488 (BEEF) + 0.145 (HDLCHM) + 0.328 (CHICKN) + 0.228 (MKWB) + 0.291 (FISHSH) + 0.211 (EGGS) + 0.468 (BUNHDH) + 17.717
Plant protein	0.062 (BREAD) + 0.195 (SOUP) + 0.063 (BEER) + 0.426 (CAKE) + 0.245 (VEGCKD) + 0.230 (BUNHDH) + 0.060 (COOKIE) + 5.391
Animal fat	0.191 (BUTTER) + 0.348 (PORKHM) + 0.289 (MKWB) + 0.167 (HDLCHM) + 0.341 (BEEF) + 0.536 (BUNHDH) + 16.465
Plant fat	0.188 (DOUNUT) + 0.680 (PIE) + 0.303 (FRDROL) + 0.547 (BUNHDH) + 0.153 (COOKIE) + 0.102 (MARG) + 0.289 (POTATO) + 0.696 (CAKE) + 5.598
Refined carbohydrate	0.759 (COKE) + 0.382 (COOKIE) + 0.104 (SUGAR) + 1.441 (PIE) + 1.875 (CAKE) + 11.484
Other carbohydrate	0.39 (BREAD) + 1.51 (VEGCKD) + 1.25 (MPLSYP) + 0.51 (BEER) + 0.61 (COOKIE) + 1.32 (CERDRY) + 1.50 (POTATO) + 0.73 (SOUP) + 47.18
Alcohol	0.326 (WHISKEY) + 0.356 (BEER) + 0.413

[a] Variables are listed in the order of entry into equations.

The relationship between number of days at modal pattern and (1) number of nutrients showing significant variation among the 12 sets (Figure 3) and (2) number of nutrients showing significant differences betwen odd and even sets of records (Figure 4) suggests independence of modal pattern and the variation in nutrients over time. Similar patterns were observed for the other comparisons of sets of records.

The results of the history interview are shown in Table 15 with the food items listed in order from the least to the highest number of differences between the recorded frequency and the history reports of frequency. Those food items also tested in the multiple regression analysis are indicated on this table. For almost all foods, subjects reported more frequent use than their records showed. The degree of consistency of history for individual items and their eventual use in the regression equations does not appear to be related.

The percent distribution of subjects by the number of significant differences between history and recorded frequency of consumption of foods is shown in Figure 5. The bimodal distribution suggests two populations of historians, one more valid than the other.

A comparison of the disagreements between history and recording both to the analysis of variance data and to the distributions of percent of days with modal patterns of eating is shown in Table 16. None of the correlation coefficients is significant.

TABLE 12 Actual Mean Daily Intake for Four Groups of Men and Women and Predicted Mean for Daily Intake

	MS Men		Executive Men		Physical Fitness Men		MS Women	
	Mean	SD	Mean	SD	Mean	SD	Mean	SD
Calories								
Actual	2,145	±530.0	2,567	±465.0	2,180	±434.0	1,694	±458.0
Predicted	2,112	±524.0	2,506	±441.0	1,974	±540.0	1,773	±404.0
Protein								
Animal								
Actual	60.8	±15.8	73.5	±14.2	71.7	±12.7	45.6	±13.7
Predicted	60.4	±15.5	70.7	±14.5	64.5	±14.9	43.5	±10.0
Plant								
Actual	21.3	±4.9	24.8	±5.2	22.7	±5.7	16.6	±4.6
Predicted	21.2	±5.1	24.0	±4.9	19.8	±5.9	17.0	±4.0
Fat								
Animal								
Actual	64.3	±22.9	67.7	±21.0	57.8	±15.2	45.4	±15.2
Predicted	63.5	±25.2	65.1	±19.8	52.5	±17.7	44.6	±12.2
Plant								
Actual	29.9	±10.7	38.2	±10.6	37.9	±14.1	28.3	±11.0
Predicted	32.5	±10.7	38.1	±11.5	40.3	±13.7	31.2	±11.4
Carbohydrate								
Refined								
Actual	59.5	±29.5	50.3	±24.4	43.7	±16.4	53.2	±22.7
Predicted	47.7	±24.2	41.6	±20.4	36.9	±16.5	43.6	±17.6
Other								
Actual	174.2	±38.7	190.1	±40.0	175.8	±35.7	137.8	±42.5
Predicted	168.1	±38.4	187.4	±35.9	151.9	±35.9	140.1	±36.2
Alcohol								
Actual	8.4	±19.7	36.3	±24.7	10.1	±9.8	4.5	±8.7
Predicted	8.7	±20.4	35.7	±24.9	11.7	±14.1	4.3	±9.5

TABLE 13 Modal Pattern for Number of Meals and/or Snacks per Day

Modal Pattern	Number of Subjects Group I—F (41)	Group I—M (32)	Group II—M (54)
3 Meals[a]	2	4	4
3 Meals + Snack 3 + 5 + 7	17	12	34
3 Meals + Snack 7	4	4	3
3 Meals + Snack 5 + 7	10	3	3
3 Meals + Snack 3 + 5	0	1	4
3 Meals + Snack 3 + 7	1	0	4
Other modal pattern[b]	7	8	2

[a] Breakfast, lunch and dinner
Snack 3—between breakfast and lunch
Snack 5—between lunch and dinner
Snack 7—after dinner
[b] Other modal patterns include any 2 or 3 meals in combination with various snacks.

TABLE 14 The Distribution of Subjects by the Percent of 36 Days That the Modal Meal Pattern Occurred

Percent of Days at Mode	Subjects No.	Percent
100	2	1.6
75–99	17	13.4
50–74	32	25.2
25–49	67	52.8
<25	9	7.1
TOTAL	127	100.0

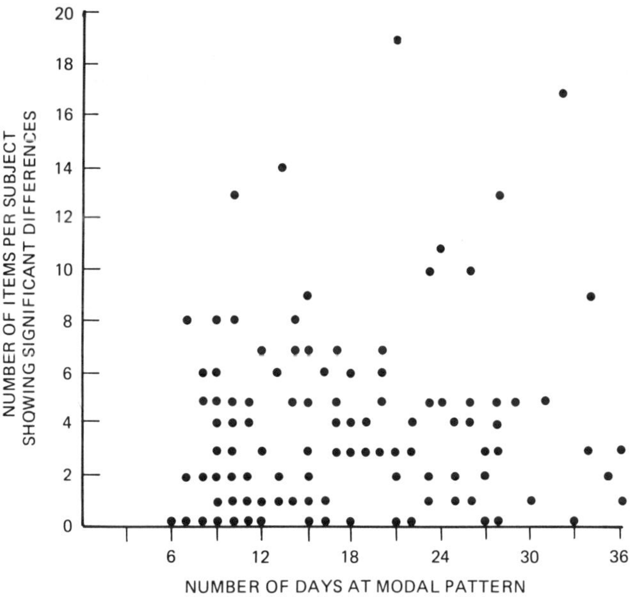

FIGURE 3 Comparison of frequency of significant differences among 12 three-day records for 19 nutrients and modal pattern.

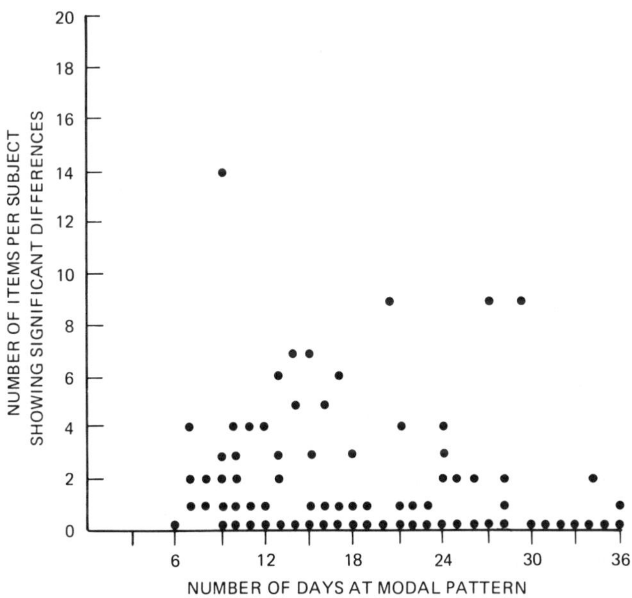

FIGURE 4 Comparison of frequency of significant differences between odd sets and even sets of records and frequency of days at modal pattern.

TABLE 15 The Occurrence of Significant Differences Between the Frequency of Consumption of Food Determined by Interview and the Recorded Frequency from 36 Days of Food Diaries in 73 Adults and the Use of the Items in Multiple Regression Analysis for Prediction of Nutrient Intake

				Tested for Prediction		
	Observed			Yes		No
Food	Less	More	Total	Used	Not Used	
Sardines, anchovies	0	0	0			x
Pizza	0	0	0			x
Waffles, pancakes	0	0	0			x
Rice	1	0	1		x	
Dry fruit	1	1	2			x
Vegetable salad	2	0	2			x
Cottage cheese	0	3	3			x
Sherbert	1	2	3			x
Bacon	1	3	4		x	
Pudding, custard	1	3	4		x	
Wine	4	0	4			x
Syrup	5	0	5	x		
Beer	5	1	6	x		
Ice cream	6	1	7		x	
Doughnuts	7	1	8	x		
Pickles, olives	2	6	8			x
Whiskey, gin	5	3	8	x		
Spaghetti, macaroni	6	3	9			x
Citrus juice	7	2	9			x
Cream soup	6	3	9	x		
Popcorn, Fritos	5	4	9		x	
Hotdog, hamburger buns	9	0	9	x		
Eggs	7	3	10	x		
Fish, shrimp	10	0	10	x		
Cooked vegetables (green, yellow)	4	6	10	x		
Cereal	7	4	11	x		
Steak, beef	3	8	11	x		
Chicken	10	1	11	x		
Potatoes	8	3	11	x		
Canned fruit	9	2	11		x	
Soup, clear	11	0	11	x		
Kool Ade, fruit ade	11	0	11		x	
Pie	11	1	12	x		
Chocolate candy	6	7	13			x
Jelly, honey	11	3	14		x	
Citrus fruit	12	2	14		x	
Other raw fruit	10	4	14		x	
Soft drinks	10	5	15	x		
Sweet rolls	10	5	15			x
Crackers	15	1	16		x	
Cheese	9	8	17		x	

TABLE 15 *Continued*

	Observed			Tested for Protection		
				Yes		No
Food	Less	More	Total	Used	Not Used	
Cream	15	2	17		x	
Gravy	11	7	18		x	
Noncitrus juices	8	10	18		x	
> 1/2 Pound meat	15	4	19	x		
Lunchmeat	3	17	20	x		
Cake, brownies	20	0	20	x		
Cookies	10	10	20	x	x	
Nonchocolate candy	11	9	20		x	
Other cooked vegetables	20	1	21	x		
Tea	22	1	23		x	

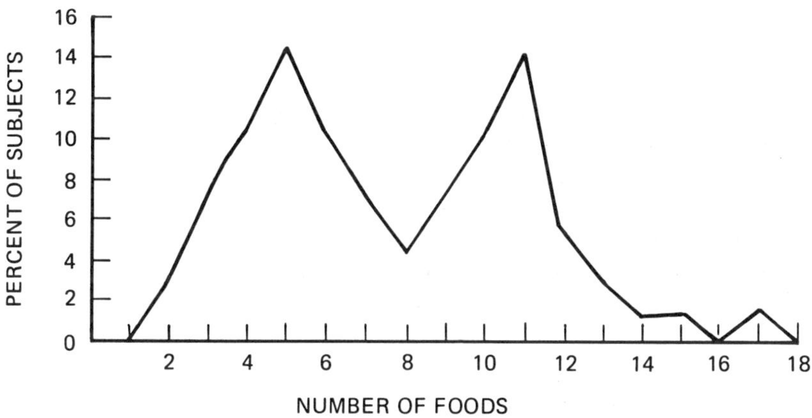

FIGURE 5 The percent distribution of 70 subjects by the number of significant differences between stated and recorded usual frequency of consumption of specific foods.

TABLE 16 Correlation Coefficients Between History and Recording Disagreements and (1) Frequency of Nutrients with Significant Variation Among 12 Sets of Records and (2) Percent of Days at Modal Pattern of Meals

	MS Men (31)			MS Women (39)		
	Significant Differences		Percent of	Significant differences		Percent of
	12 sets	History	Modal Days	12 Sets	History	Modal Days
Mean	4.77	7.87	49.3	4.15	7.67	55.8
SD	3.34	3.51	22.2	3.88	3.48	20.2
r	0.15		−0.23	−0.15		0.05

DISCUSSION

The present studies have been directed to evaluation of methods for determining the usual nutrient intake of an individual rather than the mean intake for groups of individuals. The relatively close prediction of mean intake for groups of subjects by the multiple regression equations and the relatively poor prediction by these same equations for individuals in each group, highlight the problem of determining with sufficient precision the individual intake in contrast to a group of individuals. Of course, precision is relative to the purpose for which data are collected. The analyses here have concentrated on significant difference within individuals over time and considered the relative frequency of these differences by individual nutrients or by number of differences per individual. When one considers the total possible differences, that is 21 × 127 or 2,667, for the difference in means one is struck by the relatively low percent, ranging from 3.7 to 13.4, of significant differences for the groups as a whole. However, the proportion of individuals showing mean differences is much higher when 3-day sets of records are compared by season, by alternate months, and particularly by weekdays versus weekend days. Twelve to 32 percent of subjects show significant variation for individual nutrients among the 12 sets of records at approximately monthly intervals.

It is apparent from our studies that some nutrients vary more than others and that some individuals vary more than others. Thus, the frequency of obtaining diet information is determined both by the nutrient or nutrients of interest and the proportion of individuals about whom reasonably accurate information is desired. Our studies suggest, as have others, that a representative food intake must include weekend days and weekdays, probably in their true proportion of all days. The data also suggest that a single day's information will yield data equivalent to 3 consecutive days. The data also suggest that infrequent sampling during the year, such as every other month, will provide representative information. They also suggest that sampling over a long term, such as a year, will provide more representative data than sampling over a shorter term.

The use of a limited number of food items to predict nutrient intake does not appear to be a good estimator of total intake from our data. The selection of the appropriate items is one problem. It is extremely unlikely that *a priori* selection of items by us would have included those indicated by our multiple regression equations. Translation of our items to another group is unlikely to provide good individual estimates in that group.

If information about individual foods is obtained by history, our data suggest that estimation of usual intake would be poor. Our subjects tended to overestimate their consumption of the foods used in our regression equations. Our history data also suggest that some foods are better remembered than others and that this is not related to the frequency of consumption of the foods. As with the variability of 3-day intakes, some foods are good historical items and some subjects are good historians. How to identify each is a problem.

The use of modal patterns of eating as an aid in obtaining diet histories, a technique that has proved useful in determining alcohol intake, does not appear from our data to be helpful. The proportion of days in which the modal pattern is followed is relatively low overall and those subjects with a high proportion of modal days do no better in history nor do they show less variation among their sets of records.

In summary, our data suggest that the diary recording of a single day's intake, randomly selected to represent weekdays and weekend days, with the recording done over a long enough interval to detect cyclic changes during the year resulted in a valid estimate of the usual intake of the individuals in our study. The subjects were not a probability sample of any defined population and any translation of our findings to any population would be conjectural. Further, within our study population, historical information about frequency of consumption of specific foods, knowledge of modal patterns of eating, or the use of predictive formulas for estimating nutrient intake were found wanting in their use for determination of individual dietary intake.

REFERENCES

Bebb, H. T., H. B. Houser, J. C. Witschi, A. S. Littell, and R. K. Fuller. 1971. Calorie and nutrient contribution of alcoholic beverages to the usual diets of 155 adults. Am. J. Clin. Nutr. 24:1042.

Bebb, H. T., H. B. Houser, J. C. Witschi, and A. S. Littell. 1972. Nutritive content of the usual diets of eighty-two men. J. Am. Dietet. Assoc. 61:407.

Houser, H. B., W. Insull, Jr., J. C. Vandervort, A. S. Littell, and A. I. Sorensen. 1966. The relationships of habitual diets to the fatty acid composition of adipose tissue and serum cholesterol concentration in man. Circulation 34–4: Suppl. 111–130. (Abstract)

Houser, H. B., A. I. Sorensen, A. S. Littell, and J. D. Vandervort. 1969. Dietary intake of non-hospitalized persons with multiple sclerosis. 1. Food diary and coding methods. J. Am. Dietet. Assoc. 54:391.

HVH–CWRU Nutrient Data Base. Department of Biometry, School of Medicine, Case Western Reserve University, Cleveland, Ohio.

Witschi, J. C., H. B. Houser, and A. S. Littell. 1970a. Performed vitamin A, carotene, and total vitamin A activity in usual adult diets. J. Am. Dietet. Assoc. 57:13.

Witschi, J. C., A. S. Littell, H. B. Houser, and A. I. Sorensen. 1970b. Dietary intake of non-hospitalized persons with multiple sclerosis. 2. Nutrient intake for one year compared with recommended allowances. J. Am. Dietet. Assoc. 56:203.

Diary–Interview Technique to Assess Food Consumption Patterns of Individual Military Personnel

D. D. SCHNAKENBERG, T. M. HILL,
M. J. KRETSCH, *and* B. S. MORRIS

A diary–interview technique has been developed at Letterman Army Institute of Research (LAIR) for collecting and evaluating food consumption data from individual military personnel. Under the direction of Col. John E. Canham, M.D., the technique was initially developed by Dr. Terrell M. Hill and first used at Ent Air Force Base, Colo., to measure nutrient consumption of airmen away from the dining hall (Table 1). More recently, we have used the technique to evaluate and predict the nutritional impact of new concepts of food service that are being tested at a number of Department of Defense installations.

Our diary–interview technique combines selected aspects of conventional dietary recall, food diary, and dietary interview metholologies so as to

TABLE 1 Recent Military Nutrition Studies That Have Utilized a Diary–Interview Technique to Assess the Nutrient Consumption of Individuals

Location	Date	No. of Subjects	Duration
Air Force—Ent AFB, Colo.	Oct. 1973	149	14 days
Navy—Alameda, Calif.	Mar. 1975	133	17 days
	Jun. 1976	154	14 days
	Aug. 1976	158	17 days
Marines—Twentynine Palms, Calif.	Mar. 1977	315[a]	14 days
	Oct. 1978	Ongoing	
Navy—USS *Saratoga*	Jul. 1977	203	17 days
	Nov. 1978	Ongoing	

[a] Includes 36 female marines.

hopefully optimize those unique opportunities and requirements for nutrition studies available in a military setting. Subjects who have been selected to participate in the study are briefed as to the purpose of the study, the measures used to maintain the confidentiality of individual data, what will be expected of them as participants, and where and when to report for the series of 20-minute meetings with one of our interviewers. At the first meeting, the subject is asked to recall all foods (except spices) and beverages (except water) consumed during the previous day. The subject is instructed to itemize the information on a pocket-sized card (Figure 1) and to also record the time the item was consumed, the quantity consumed, and the source of each item (e.g., military dining hall, home, restaurant, or vendor). The participant is provided this card as a guide to record food consumption on identical diary cards for the next 3 to 4 days. At the subsequent twice-

DAILY FOOD CONSUMPTION

NAME ____________________ SUBJ. NO. __________

SSAN ____________________ DATE __________

TIME	FOOD ITEM	AMOUNT	SC

LAIR FORM 43 (4 Feb 75 - Bioenergetics)

FIGURE 1 Daily food consumption.

weekly interviews, the diary cards are returned to the interviewer for review, assistance in estimating portion size, clarification of any unusual food items consumed, and assignment of each food item as a component of either a meal or a between-meal snack.

In most of our studies, we have hired female dietitians and public health nutritionists, on a temporary basis, to serve as interviewers and to code and verify the data for subsequent computer processing. We did, however, train and use male military and civil service biological laboratory technicians as interviewers for the study conducted aboard the aircraft carrier USS *Saratoga,* while on station in the Mediterranean Sea.

The March 1975 study at Naval Air Station, Alameda, Calif., provided an opportunity to assess the validity of our diary–interview technique to estimate nutrient intake per dining hall meal (Table 2).

As a separate aspect of the survey, we stationed additional dietitians at the end of each serving line in the dining hall who recorded, by observation, the food items selected by each and every patron of the dining hall. Portion size was determined by weighing the total quantity served and dividing it by the number of portions taken. The food waste on each tray was weighed and subtracted from serving size to obtain the amount consumed. The last four digits of the social security numbers were used to track the trays of all individual patrons and to identify the diary–interview participants. Upon examination of both the diary–interview and observer data bases, we found 423 man-days where the number of reported and observed meals agreed and

TABLE 2 Nutrition Survey, Naval Air Station, Alameda, Calif., March 1975

	Technique	
	Daily Diary–Dietary Interview	Observer
Purpose	Total daily intake	Intake per dining hall meal
Length of study	17 days	17 days
Population studied	133	All
Weight of food item consumed	As reported	Average portion size minus individual plate waste
Composition of foods consumed	Nutrient factor file	Nutrient factor file
Man-days test population utilized dining hall	534	458
Man-days number of reported and observed meals agreed	423	423
Number of subjects	62	62

these man-days of data were derived from 62 of the 133 subjects in the test population. The same nutrient factor file of food composition tables was used in the computation of both data bases.

One variable in the comparison of the two techniques was the relative agreement in food item selection (Table 3). Food items selected agreed between the two techniques 80 percent of the time. Fourteen percent of the total food items in question were observed but not reported to have been consumed. Only 6 percent of items were reported but not observed. The relative incidence of disagreements by food type are also shown in Table 3. Vegetables, fruits, nuts, and legumes were included in the other food type category.

The average nutrient intake per dining hall meal was computed for each of the 62 subjects utilizing the data derived from the two techniques and the comparisons are shown on Table 4. With the exception of protein, fat, and niacin, which did not differ, the diary–interview method significantly underestimated nutrient intake per meal compared to the observer technique. However, the magnitude of the underestimation was usually 10 percent or less. The lower values for the interview technique reflect, in part, the previously mentioned greater tendency for an individual to have been observed to consume a food but not report it on his diary card. The larger discrepancy in ascorbic acid intake (41.2 mg vs. 58.0 mg/meal) is partially artifactitious. If an

TABLE 3 Comparison of Diary–Interview and Observer Techniques to Assess Food Item Consumption per Dining Hall Meal, Naval Air Station, Alameda, Calif., March 1975

	Number of Food Items per Meal		
	Mean	SD	Range
Foods in question[a]	6.51[b]	1.66	2–12
Foods in agreement	5.20	1.73	0–12
Foods reported but not observed	0.42	0.73	0–5
Foods observed but not reported	0.89	0.95	0–4
Disagreements in entrees	0.20	0.47	0–3
Disagreements in salads	0.11	0.29	0–2
Disagreements in desserts	0.15	0.40	0–2
Disagreements in beverages	0.20	0.41	0–2
Disagreements in other food types	0.65	0.81	0–4
Ratio of agreements to total foods in question			0.80
Ratio of reported but not observed to total foods in question			0.06
Ratio of observed but not reported to total foods in question			0.14

[a]Condiments excluded.
[b]n = 423 man-days.

TABLE 4 Comparison of Diary–Interview and Observer Techniques to Estimate Nutrient Intake per Dining Hall Meal, Naval Air Station, Alameda, Calif., March 1975

	Technique[a]		
Nutrient	Diary–Interview	Observer	P Value[b]
Quantity, g	917 ± 253[c]	1,042 ± 288[c]	<0.001
Energy, g	1,237 ± 354	1,373 ± 362	<0.001
Protein, g	55 ± 16	57 ± 15	NS
Fat, g	62 ± 19	65 ± 18	NS
Carbohydrate, g	117 ± 42	144 ± 46	<0.001
Calcium, mg	673 ± 311	751 ± 315	0.006
Phosphorus, mg	930 ± 294	986 ± 296	0.064
Iron, mg	7.9 ± 2.1	8.8 ± 2.5	<0.001
Vitamin A, IU	2,933 ± 2,122	3,669 ± 2,385	<0.001
Thiamin, mg	0.75 ± 0.22	0.82 ± 0.22	0.022
Riboflavin, mg	1.39 ± 0.47	1.52 ± 0.50	0.010
Niacin, mg	8.67 ± 2.9	9.00 ± 3.4	NS
Ascorbic acid, mg	41.2 ± 33	58.0 ± 47	<0.001

[a] Values computed from the average nutrient intake per dining hall meal of each subject (n = 62) who reported and was observed to have utilized the dining hall one or more times during the survey.

[b] Paired t-test.

[c] Mean ± SD.

individual selected an orange but did not eat it until after leaving the dining hall, the observer technique considered it to be consumed with the meal, whereas the diary–interview technique considered it to be part of an after-meal snack.

To further examine the data, we computed a comparison ratio for each subject where:

$$\text{Comparison Ratio} = \frac{\text{Nutrient intake/meal from diary–interview technique}}{\text{Nutrient intake/meal from observer technique}}$$

As shown in Table 5, the mean comparison ratio for energy was 0.92, indicating that compared to the observer technique the diary–interview technique underestimated energy intake of the population by an average of only 8 percent. This compares favorably to the 16 percent underestimation of actual (unobtrusively weighed) energy intake per meal obtained from elderly subjects by a 7-day dietary record technique as reported by Gersovitz *et al.* (1978). However, it should also be noted that our diary–interview underestimated the energy intake of 72.6 percent of the individuals at least to some degree. The histogram of comparison ratios for energy intake is shown in Figure 2. The distribution is skewed to the left of 1.0 with 34

TABLE 5 Evaluation of Daily Diary–Interview Technique, Naval Air Station, Alameda, Calif., March 1975

	Comparison Ratios [a]		
Nutrient	Mean ± SD	Percent <1.0[b]	Percent >1.0[c]
Quantity	0.92 ± 0.30[d]	71.0	29.0
Energy	0.92 ± 0.26	72.6	27.4
Protein	1.01 ± 0.32	54.8	45.2
Fat	0.98 ± 0.28	61.3	38.7
Carbohydrate	0.85 ± 0.32	82.3	17.7
Calcium	0.96 ± 0.56	72.6	27.4
Phosphorus	1.00 ± 0.44	62.9	37.1
Iron	0.93 ± 0.26	67.7	32.3
Vitamin A	0.85 ± 0.33	75.8	24.2
Thiamin	0.96 ± 0.35	61.3	38.7
Riboflavin	0.98 ± 0.48	69.4	30.6
Niacin	1.05 ± 0.52	56.5	43.5
Ascorbic acid	0.78 ± 0.42	79.0	21.0
All variables ($\bar{x}$)	0.94	68.2	31.8

[a] Diary–interview nutrient intake ÷ observed nutrient intake.
[b] Comparison ratio less than 1.0 (diary–interview < observed).
[c] Comparison ratio greater than 1.0 (diary–interview > observed).
[d] n = 62 subjects.

percent of population in the range of 10–20 percent underestimation (comparison ratio, 0.8–0.9) of energy intake. Furthermore, 13 percent of the population underestimated by more than 30 percent and 5 percent overestimated energy intake by more than 30 percent.

Projection of the results of these dining hall meals to the evaluation of total daily nutrient intake data obtained by the same diary–interview technique is tenuous. The average total daily energy intake measured by diary–interview was 2,650 kcal, a value approximately 12 percent less than a reasonable estimate of 3,000 kcal energy expenditure for a light activity male population with an average age of 26 years and weighing an average of 76 kg. This suggests that the underestimation of energy intake away from the dining hall was greater than 10 percent.

We were concerned that the apparent greater underestimation of energy intake away from the dining hall might be due to the greater uncertainties regarding portion and unit size than in the dining hall. We have always obtained serving size information from the military dining halls and have made it available to the interviewers to use as a guide in assisting their subjects in estimating amounts consumed. At Twentynine Palms, Calif., the number of commercial food outlets readily available to the marines on and off the base is very limited. Therefore, the interviewers were able to visit

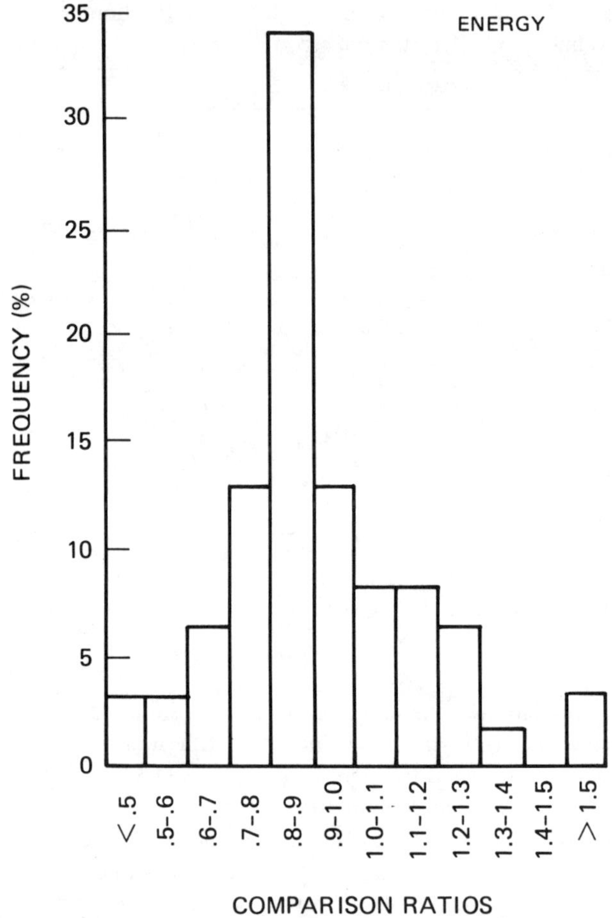

FIGURE 2

almost all of the eating establishments frequented by the marines as well as the local grocery stores and obtain portion and unit size information. The average daily energy intakes over the 14-day study period are shown in Table 6. At this time, we are unsure if we shoud attribute the nearly 500 kcal/day difference in reported energy intake between single and married male marines to group differences in reliability of data collection, to real differences in energy expenditures, or both. Since the married males consumed 82.6 percent of their calories at home compared to only 18.1 percent for the single males, even a modest bias towards greater underestimation of intake at home compared to dining halls, restaurants, and vendors would significantly

TABLE 6 Energy Intakes and Selected Demographic and Anthropometric Characteristics of Three Populations of Marines, Twentynine Palms, Calif., 1977

	Single Males	Married Males	Single Females
Number of subjects	57	59	36
Daily energy intake, kcal/day	3,105 ± 688[a]	2,637 ± 684	1,991 ± 659
Age, yr	20.5 ± 1.6	24.4 ± 5.1	20.9 ± 2.3
Height, cm	178.4 ± 7.2	176.7 ± 6.1	165.6 ± 6.4
Weight, kg	73.1 ± 8.7	76.6 ± 11.4	58.5 ± 6.9
Percent average daily energy from:			
Dining halls	52.1 ± 23.0	3.3 ± 7.7	22.1 ± 24.3
Home	18.1 ± 19.1	82.6 ± 14.2	39.1 ± 29.8
Restaurants	19.1 ± 16.1	8.0 ± 9.8	23.8 ± 17.0
Vendors	10.7 ± 9.2	6.1 ± 7.2	15.0 ± 12.3

[a]Mean ± SD.

contribute to the reported differences in total daily energy intake. During the current study at Twentynine Palms, we are asking some of the diary–interview subjects to wear heart-rate monitors during 24 to 72 hours of the data collection period. Energy expenditure will be estimated from the average daily heart rate and an individualized heart rate versus oxygen consumption curve obtained during a graded exercise test. We are hopeful that the energy expenditure measurements, combined with weight change data, will greatly assist in our estimation of error in measuring energy intake of male and female military populations.

Our rationale for asking our subjects to maintain their food diaries for 14–17 consecutive days was to look for possible effects of weekends and payday on total daily nutrient intake. However, as shown in Figure 3, our analyses of these effects have been confounded by a definite trend, especially in the male subjects, to report consuming fewer calories as the duration of the study was extended. For example, at Twentynine Palms the single males reported consuming almost 3,400 kcal/day during the first 3 days, compared to approximately 2,900 kcal/day during the last 3 days of the 14-day study (Figure 3). The magnitude of the decline was approximately 200 kcal/day for the female marines. The decline in reported intake may reflect a change in attitude of many of the subjects as the novelty of the study wears off and they begin to tire of maintaining the diary record. Dr. Kretsch is currently analyzing these data to try to select the appropriate duration for our studies and is also comparing these diary–interview data to the dietary recall data we obtained during the first visit with the subjects.

During the USS *Saratoga* study, we obtained 21-day body-weight change data in addition to age, weight, height, skinfold thicknesses, and perceived

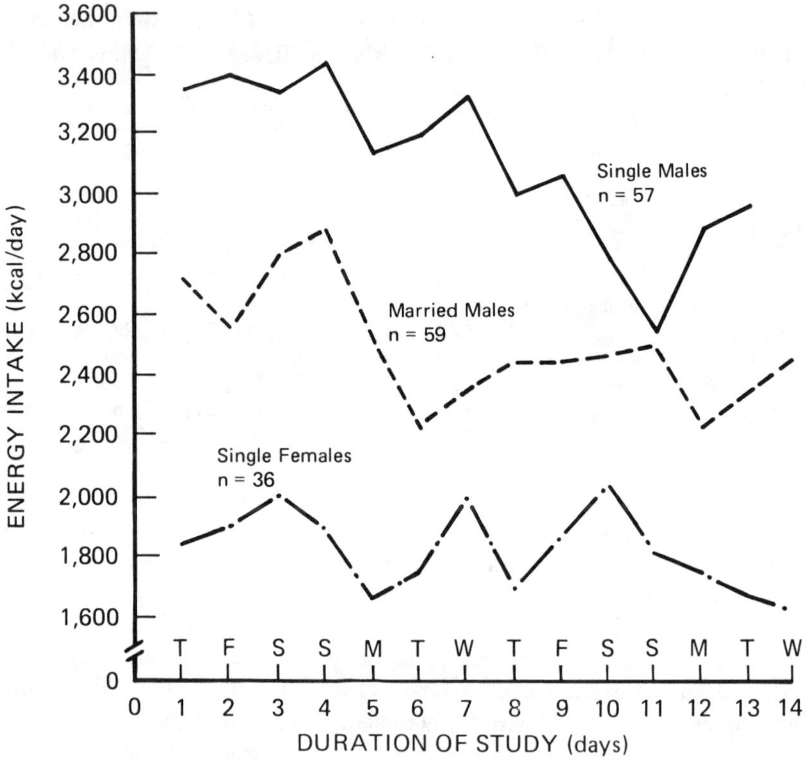

FIGURE 3

level of physical activity (light, moderate, heavy) information. These data were used to compute a predicted daily energy expenditure value for each subject. A reliability index value was computed for each subject by the following:

$$\text{Reliability Index} = \frac{\text{Reported daily energy intake}}{\text{Predicted daily energy expenditure}}$$

For the entire population, the reported daily energy intake over the 17-day period was 2,004 kcal/day, compared to a predicted daily energy expenditure of 3,040 kcal/day. To try to determine why the reported energy intakes were so much lower than in previous studies, Dr. Schnakenberg used the Reliability Index to divide the population into "more reliable subjects" (index $\geqslant$0.8) and "less reliable subjects" (index <0.8). As shown in Figure 4, the reported total daily energy intakes dropped precipitously during the first 7 days

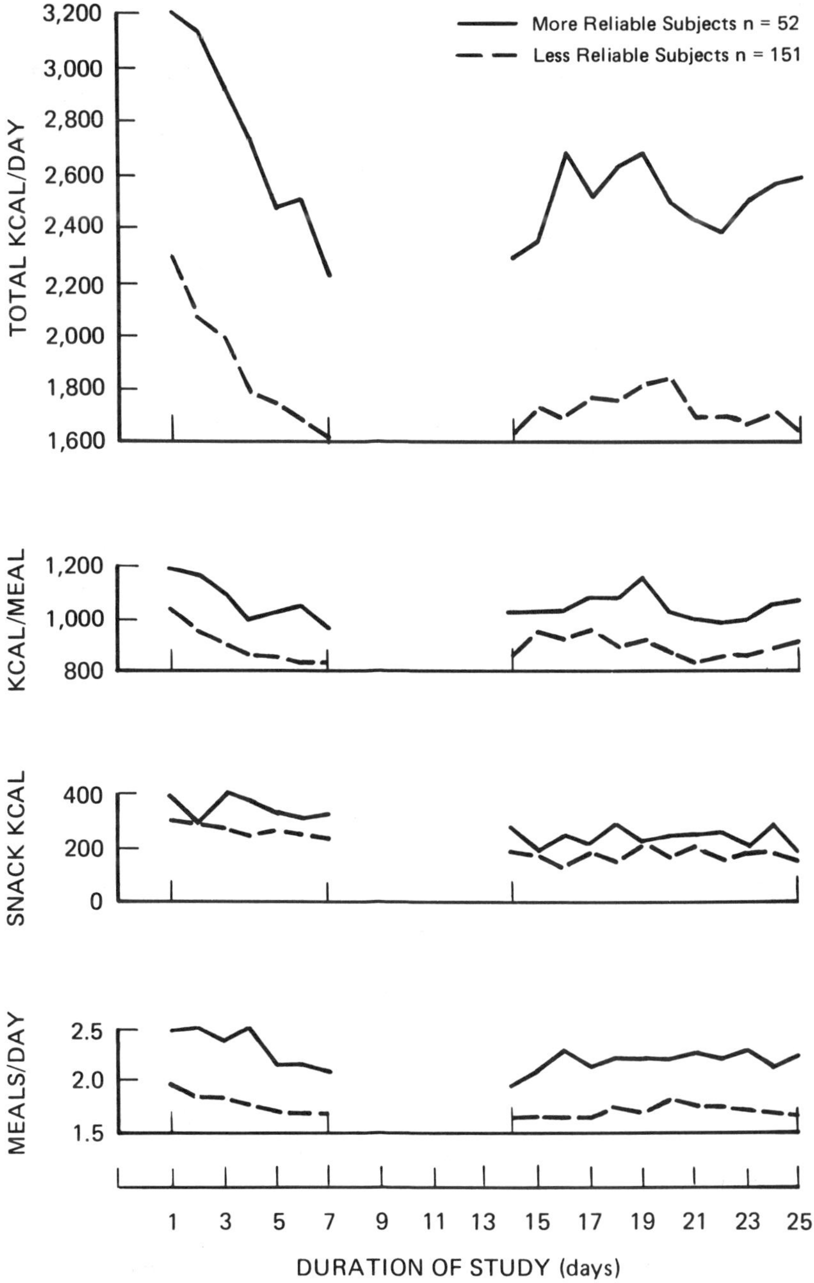
More Reliable Subjects n = 52
Less Reliable Subjects n = 151
TOTAL KCAL/DAY
3,200
3,000
2,800
2,600
2,400
2,200
2,000
1,800
1,600
KCAL/MEAL
1,200
1,000
800
SNACK KCAL
400
200
0
MEALS/DAY
2.5
2.0
1.5
1 3 5 7 9 11 13 15 17 19 21 23 25
DURATION OF STUDY (days)

FIGURE 4

of the study. Following an 8-day in-port period when data were not collected, reported energy intake stabilized at a low level. The 50–100 kcal/day drop in reported calories from snacks contributed only slightly to the 600–700 kcal decline in total daily energy intake. Therefore, the major factors were the decline in kcal/meal and the reduced number of meals reported being consumed per day. It is interesting to note that the curves of the "more reliable" and "less reliable" subjects are essentially parallel. We conducted this study at the beginning of the 7-month long cruise, and the subjects' adjustments to the rigors of sea duty and separation from family and friends may have contributed to the problems in completeness of data collection.

The *Saratoga* study posed a serious problem for data evaluation and interpretation. Despite the conscientious efforts of all members of the survey team, the data collection procedures resulted in the average energy intake of the population being underestimated by approximately 30–35 percent. Therefore, should the data of only those subjects whose energy intakes appear to be reasonably complete be used in the evaluation of the food service system or should all the subjects be included? If an estimate of the number of lunch meals consumed in the forward galley was needed by food service delivery system planners, Dr. Schnakenberg used data from only the more reliable subjects. However, he used data from all subjects to evaluate the nutritional adequacy of meals and total diet consumed on the ship. This was because of concern that the more reliable subjects might have a greater nutritional awareness and better food selection patterns than their less reliable counterparts. He has assumed however, that although incomplete, the reported nutrient intakes of the less reliable subjects are a representative sample of their food selection patterns. With this assumption, he expressed the nutrient intake data on essentially a nutrient density basis by using the concept of Nutrient Ratio (NR), where:

$$\text{NR} = \frac{\text{Intake expressed per 1,000 kcal consumed}}{\text{Nutritional standard expressed per 1,000 kcal}}$$

He further tried to simplify the data evaluation process by categorizing the nutrient intakes as either "low," "marginal," or "adequate" according to the following arbitrarily selected criteria:

"Low" (NR <0.7) intake less than 70 percent of standard
"Marginal" (NR $0.7 <1.0$) intake between 70 percent and 100 percent of standard
"Adequate" (NR≥ 1.0) intake greater than 100 percent of standard

The military dietary allowances (Departments of the Army, the Navy, and the Air Force, 1976) were used as the nutritional standards for these calculations.

The nutrient ratio concept can be used not only to evaluate the adequacy of average daily nutrient intakes (Table 7), but also to compare the nutritional adequacy of meals consumed from various sources such as the aft galley (Table 8), forward galley (Table 9), and nongalley nutrition (Table 10) and to monitor the eating habits (Table 11) and food type consumption patterns (Table 12) of individuals with low, marginal, or adequate intakes of specific nutrients. This type of data presentation is useful in evaluating the reasons for a high incidence of low intakes of a specific nutrient, such as

TABLE 7 Evaluation of Average Daily Nutrient Intakes, USS *Saratoga*, July–August 1977

	Percentage of Population [a]		
Nutrient	Low[b]	Marginal[c]	Adequate[d]
Protein	0	3.9	96.1
Calcium	1.5	21.2	77.3
Iron	3.0	52.7	44.3
Vitamin A	20.2	31.0	48.8
Thiamin	3.0	52.7	44.3
Riboflavin	0.5	24.1	75.4
Niacin	0.5	23.2	76.4
Vitamin C	8.4	18.2	73.4

[a] 203 subjects.
[b] Nutrient ratio <0.7.
[c] Nutrient ratio 0.7 to <1.0.
[d] Nutrient ratio ≥ 1.0.

TABLE 8 Evaluation of Aft Galley Meals, USS *Saratoga*, July–August 1977

	Percentage of Population [a]		
Nutrient	Low[b]	Marginal[c]	Adequate[d]
Protein	0	0	100
Calcium	5.4	19.8	74.8
Iron	0.5	28.2	71.3
Vitamin A	10.4	22.8	66.8
Thiamin	0.5	33.2	66.3
Riboflavin	0	10.9	89.1
Niacin	0	9.9	90.1
Vitamin C	5.0	9.9	85.1

[a] 202 subjects who reported eating at least one meal in aft galley.
[b] Nutrient ratio <0.7.
[c] Nutrient ratio 0.7 to <1.0.
[d] Nutrient ratio ≥ 1.0.

TABLE 9 Evaluation of Forward Galley Meals, USS *Saratoga*, July–August 1977

	Percentage of Population [a]		
Nutrient	Low[b]	Marginal[c]	Adequate[d]
Protein	0.5	13.0	86.4
Calcium	7.1	17.9	75.0
Iron	8.7	43.5	47.8
Vitamin A	61.4	26.1	12.5
Thiamin	2.2	39.1	58.7
Riboflavin	1.1	32.6	66.3
Niacin	8.2	31.5	60.3
Vitamin C	50.0	14.1	35.9

[a] 184 subjects who reported eating at least one meal in forward galley.
[b] Nutrient ratio <0.7.
[c] Nutrient ratio 0.7 to <1.0.
[d] Nutrient ratio ≥ 1.0.

TABLE 10 Evaluation of Nongalley Nutrition, USS *Saratoga*, July–August 1977

	Percentage of Population[a]		
Nutrient	Low[b]	Marginal[c]	Adequate[d]
Protein	78.6	14.3	7.1
Calcium	19.4	38.3	42.3
Iron	76.0	10.7	13.3
Vitamin A	91.3	3.6	5.1
Thiamin	89.3	6.1	4.6
Riboflavin	73.5	8.2	18.4
Niacin	68.4	6.6	25.0
Vitamin C	77.0	3.6	19.4

[a] 196 subjects who reported consuming foods and beverages from sources other than from aft and forward galley meals.
[b] Nutrient ratio <0.7.
[c] Nutrient ratio 0.7 to <1.0.
[d] Nutrient ratio ≥ 1.0.

vitamin A, and in designing and predicting the impact of intervention programs. For example, 61 percent of the meals consumed in the forward galley (Table 9) were low in vitamin A, indicating that a salad bar should be added to the predominantly short order type of menu. However, because subjects with low vitamin A intakes (Table 12) avoid tomatoes, carrots, leafy and green vegetables, it is unlikely that simply adding a salad bar will markedly increase the vitamin A intakes of this group. As shown in Table 11, the low vitamin A intake group selected meals from the aft galley that were low in vitamin A (NR =0.73), even though vitamin A was abundantly available.

TABLE 11 Comparison of Eating Habits of Subjects with Low, Marginal, or Adequate Daily Vitamin A Intakes, USS *Saratoga*, July – August 1977

	All Subjects	Subjects Whose Daily Vitamin Intakes Were:		
		Low[a]	Marginal[b]	Adequate[c]
No. of subjects	203	41	63	99
No. aft galley meals/day	1.50 ± .58[d]	1.10 ± .57[d]	1.47 ± .59[d]	1.68 ± .49[d]
No. elsewhere meals/day	0.40 ± .34	0.55 ± .34	0.43 ± .36	0.31 ± .29
No. total meals/day	1.89 ± .52	1.65 ± .52	1.90 ± .54	1.99 ± .47
% of kcal from aft meals	68.0 ± 19.7	52.2 ± 22.2	66.6 ± 17.4	75.5 ± 15.7
% of kcal from forward meals	18.0 ± 15.2	25.3 ± 16.1	20.1 ± 15.8	13.6 ± 12.9
% of kcal from elsewhere	14.0 ± 12.2	22.5 ± 16.6	13.3 ± 10.7	10.9 ± 8.9
% of kcal from snacks	12.4 ± 10.5	19.3 ± 13.7	11.8 ± 9.0	10.0 ± 8.7
Vitamin A ratio				
Aft meals	1.44 ± .81	0.73 ± .16	1.06 ± .21	1.97 ± .84
Forward meals	0.70 ± .42	0.57 ± .22	0.69 ± .32	0.77 ± .52
Nutrition obtained elsewhere	0.28 ± .40	0.18 ± .18	0.26 ± .35	0.34 ± .49

[a] Vitamin A nutrient ratio <0.7.
[b] Vitamin A nutrient ratio 0.7 to <1.0.
[c] Vitamin A nutrient ratio ≥1.0.
[d] Mean ± SD for number of subjects indicated.

At sea, there is insufficient refrigerated storage space to keep fresh milk available for periods of more than 4–7 days. This problem is described in Figure 5a, where the ship ran out of fresh milk on July 15, was resupplied

TABLE 12 Food-Type Consumption of Subjects with Low, Marginal, or Adequate Vitamin A Intakes, USS *Saratoga*, July–August 1977

	Quantity (g/day) Consumed by Subjects Whose Daily Vitamin A Intakes Were:		
	Low[a]	Marginal[b]	Adequate[c]
No. of subjects	41	63	99
Milk	137	236	178
Cheeses and ice cream	19	29	31
Tomatoes and tomato products	9	25	38
Carrots, raw and cooked	0.2	1.5	8
Sweet potatoes	0.3	1.8	2.0
Liver	0	0	1.3
Leafy and green vegetables	6	14	31
Melons, peaches, plums	11	12	28
Eggs	24	41	42
Potatoes, french fries	8	11	11

[a]Nutrient ratio <0.7.
[b]Nutrient ratio 0.7 to <1.0.
[c]Nutrient ratio ≥1.0.

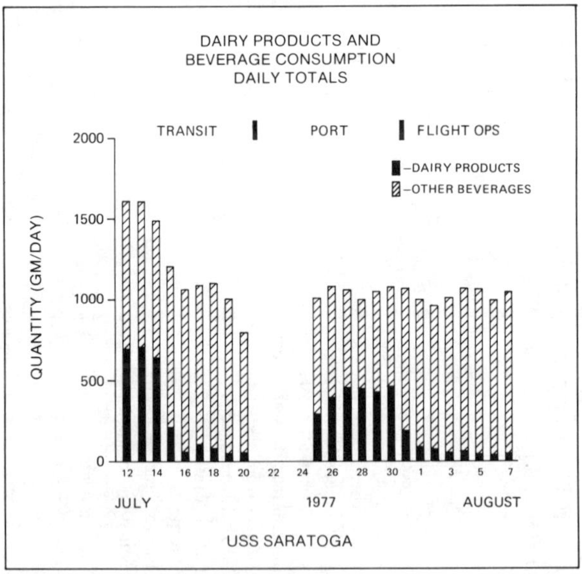

FIGURE 5a

with filled milk while in port, and ran out again on July 31. The consumption of carbonated and noncarbonated beverages markedly increased when milk was not available. The percentage of the population with low and marginal intakes of calcium (Figure 5b) and riboflavin (Figure 5c) substantially increased on days when milk was not available. At our urging, a low-fat (25–30 percent fat calories) vitamin A-fortified (30 percent RDA per

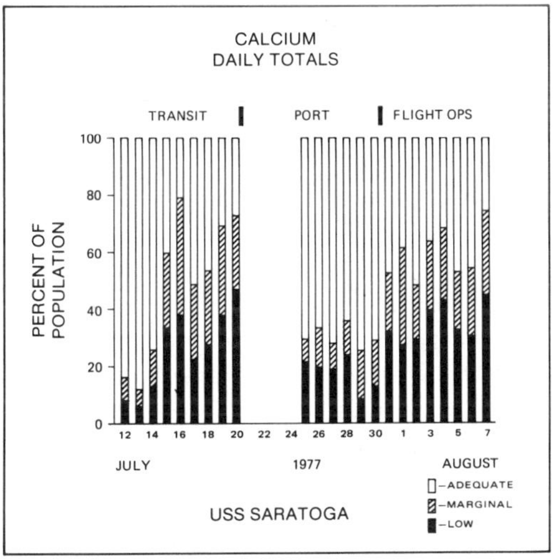

FIGURE 5b

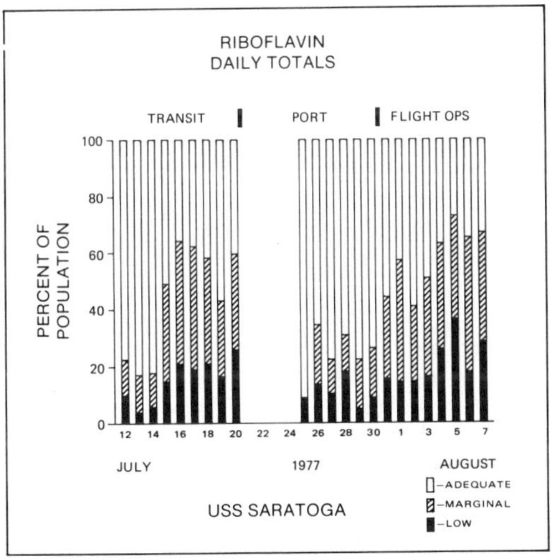

FIGURE 5c

serving) milk shake, which is reconstituted aboard ship from a dry shelf stable base, is being tested on the USS *Saratoga*. Based upon the food-type selection patterns previously shown in Table 12, we have projected that this product will effectively reduce the incidence of low and marginal intakes of calcium, riboflavin, and vitamin A as shown in Table 13. One of the primary purposes of our current follow-up study on the USS *Saratoga* is to assess the validity of our projections.

As a result of our recent experiences from seven dietary assessment studies in a variety of military settings and our attempts to validate our methodology, we have made some modifications to our dietary–interview technique. Most significantly, we have reduced the time the participants are asked to maintain their food diaries from 14–17 days to no more than 7–8 consecutive days. We believe that 7–8 days is long enough to obtain a reliable sample of an individual's eating patterns and food selection habits, but short enough to maintain a cooperative attitude in most of the participants. It is still essential though that a diary review session be scheduled 3–4 days after the initial interview. We are incorporating some sort of validation procedures in each of our studies, most of which focus on obtaining an estimate of the energy expenditure level of each subject. However, we are keenly aware that the magnitude of the error in estimation of energy expen-

TABLE 13 Projected Nutritional Impact of Offering Vitamin A-Enriched Milk Shakes,[a] USS *Saratoga*

	Percentage of Population		
Nutrient	Low	Marginal	Adequate
Calcium intake			
Jul.–Aug. 1977	2	21	77
Projected[b]	2	10	88
Riboflavin intake			
Jul.–Aug. 1977	1	24	75
Projected[b]	1	11	88
Vitamin A intake			
Jul.–Aug. 1977	20	31	49
Projected[b, c]	5	13	82

[a] Shake mix enriched to provide 1,800 IU vitamin A per 12.5 fl. oz. serving.

[b] Projections based upon Jul.–Aug. 1977 data selecting only the days when milk was available.

[c] Based upon presumption that individuals who consumed at least one glass of milk per day when available will consume one enriched milk shake per day.

NOTE: These projections assumed that milk shakes will be available at both forward and aft galleys.

diture and short-term caloric deficit or surfeit of individuals may be as large as the error in estimating energy consumption. Therefore, we are beginning to concentrate more on utilizing a nutrient ratio, nutrient balance, or, if you prefer, nutrient density approach to the analysis and interpretation of the data rather than limiting our interpretations to reported average daily quantities of nutrients consumed. We are rapidly expanding our computer programming capabilities so that we can more fully utilize the information contained in our data bank. Mr. Morris has developed the necessary software to retrieve individual nutrient intake data by demographic and anthropometric characteristics, by date, by time (breakfast, lunch, supper, etc.), by source (home, restaurant, vendor, dining hall, etc.), or by combination of several variables. We can also retrieve, by individual or group, the quantity of any food item (limited to the ~2,500 different food items currently on our Nutrient Factor File), or food type consumed. Dr. Kretsch has recently overseen the addition of cholesterol, animal/plant protein, and animal/plant/marine fat values for nearly all food items on the file and a significant number of vitamin E, vitamin B_6, vitamin B_{12}, folic acid, magnesium, copper, zinc, manganese, pantothenic acid, and fatty acids values have been added. These improvements in our data-processing and retrieval system should significantly contribute to the knowledge base of nutrient intake patterns of not only military personnel but our young adult population in general.

REFERENCES

Departments of the Army, the Navy, and the Air Force. 1976. Army Regulation 40-25, BUMED Instruction 10110.3E, and Air Force Regulation 160-95. Medical services nutritional standards. Departments of the Army, the Navy, and the Air Force, Washington, D.C., 30 August 1976 (as corrected).

Gersovitz, M., J. P. Madden, and H. Smiciklas-Wright. 1978. Validity of the 24-hr. dietary recall and seven-day record for group comparisons. J. Am. Diet. Assoc. 73:48.

Possible Alternative Methods for Data Collection on Food Consumption and Expenditures

ROBERT B. PEARL

There are few behavioral patterns in our society that are more extensively documented than the purchase and consumption of food products. Countless practitioners, both inside and outside of government, are engaged in producing statistics on this subject either on a continuous or intermittent basis. Moreover, there are probably almost as many different methodologies and techniques employed in gathering these data as there are participants in the field.

In view of these facts, it would be surprising if almost every possible means of developing these statistics had not already been attempted or at least considered. This likelihood poses a problem for anyone charged with presenting challenging and innovative ideas along these lines. The temptation exists to opt for exotic possibilities, such as using spy satellites to chart the eating behavior of the population. The writer intends to resist this temptation in favor of a few notions that, if not entirely novel, at least do not appear to have entered the mainstream of statistical endeavors in this sector. In the main, these will be aimed at some of the principal deficiencies that are believed to exist in nutritional and dietary data.

INTERMITTENT PANELS

One of the limitations of the methodologies customarily employed in studies of food consumption is the relatively short period of observation. Because of cooperation problems and concern about reporting errors, comprehensive family consumption data have usually been restricted to a period of 1 week or less and individual intake data to a span of a very few days. Even food purchase or expenditure information has rarely been collected for more than a 2- to 4-week period.

Assuming samples of sufficient size that are adequately distributed over time, these restrictions should not impair such measures as *average* family or individual consumption. The limitation arises when an effort is made to provide *distributions* of families and persons by nutritional status. Since studies have indicated that dietary inadequacies exist in every socioeconomic group, the focus may be more on distributions and individual differences than on group averages. In view of the variations that are likely to occur in food consumption from day to day, week to week, or season to season, it is difficult to see how observation for only a brief period can validly depict the nutritional status of any one family or person.

The preferable course would probably be to observe each subject for an extensive, continuous period, perhaps up to a year. Unfortunately, experience has indicated that samples used for continuous expenditure surveys become highly biased because of attrition (Quackenbush and Shaffer, 1960), and there would be even less hope for success in the case of individual food consumption measurement. One alternative would be to attempt an intermittent panel procedure, whereby the same subjects would be canvassed at various points of the year, but for a relatively brief period each time. The data from the various observations would be accumulated to provide the measure of nutritional status. Although some further experimentation might be needed, a canvass once each quarter could be adequate for a particular case. Some analyses have indicated that a 3-week period of observation each time for family consumption might be the optimum in this type of design, balancing the need for stable measurements against that of avoiding undue sample attrition or fatigue (Ferber and Sudman, 1971; Report and Recommendations, 1976). For a specific family, the observation period could be randomly scheduled to occur at different times each quarter in order to cover a greater variety of situations.

The designation of a 3-week observation period would probably permit the use of a food purchase approach in data collection, in lieu of the more complex food consumption procedure, since the two are likely to balance out for periods of that length (especially where there would be four quarterly observations to aggregate). A food purchase approach, in turn, would likely entail the use of diary keeping, which has been found to be relatively successful for that purpose (Pearl, 1977, 1978). For individuals as opposed to families, the procedure would probably call for maintaining records of consumption for possibly a 3-day period randomized within each 3-week cycle; the family data could then be used as a control (for home consumption) over the individual data.

The use of a panel always raises problems of securing adequate cooperation over time. An appropriate incentive system might well be necessary, with a modest reward for completing any one quarterly effort and a sizeable bonus for persisting through the entire cycle. Since panel members could move from quarter to quarter, some follow-ups would be required each time, but these are not likely to exceed 5 percent of the total at any one point.

UNIVERSAL PRODUCT CODES

Another deficiency in much of the information that has been collected in this field, whether through diaries or interviews, has been inadequate and inconsistent descriptions of products. This problem is especially acute where conversion to a nutrient basis is the objective. The proliferation of prepared foods, containing a variety of ingredients, obviously adds to the difficulty.

One possible way of reducing this problem would be to make use of the Universal Product Codes (UPC) that now appear on nearly all canned and packaged food products and even on some fresh items that are repackaged in stores. Experimentation would be needed to determine whether survey respondents could be induced to enter these codes in diaries, in addition to a brief product description, and, moreover, whether they could do so accurately. If this could be achieved, and assuming that the necessary data on ingredients could be obtained from the respective manufacturers and stored in computers, conversion to a nutrient basis could become a routine matter. Moreover, consistency and reliability in reporting would be materially advanced and clerical coding and processing costs could be minimized.

AUTOMATED CHECKOUT INFORMATION

Another technological development of major interest, still limited in scope but offering promise for the future, is the appearance of automated checkout systems in food stores based on the Universal Product Codes. As these become more prevalent, they could serve as the basis for obtaining current food sales data in a level of detail never before contemplated. Although sales data are of only limited value for purposes of measuring family or individual food consumption, they could supply control totals for usually deficient survey data or at least provide a standard for evaluating survey results. Moreover, if all purchases are made by credit card in some imaginable future era, the combination of the sales data from mechanized systems and the personal characteristics of credit card holders in the possession of various financial agencies could produce the best of all possible statistical worlds. (This target may sound like "1984," but is not likely to occur by that date.)

Perhaps a more realistic application would be the use for survey purposes of the individual cash register tapes produced by the automated systems, which generally provide a far more adequate description of the products purchased than has heretofore been available. These tapes could serve as a basic reminder to survey respondents in filling diaries or responding in interviews and, in some cases, could even serve as a substitute for completing parts of diaries.

PORTABLE TAPE RECORDERS

No matter how carefully surveys of this kind are planned, serious reporting errors are likely to occur because of memory biases, tedium in filling diaries, and other reasons. A possible aid in overcoming these deficiencies would be to provide respondents with small, pocket-size tape recorders to use during the survey period. Respondents would then be asked to record purchases as they are made in the store or are being unpacked at home (possibly including UPC numbers) or, alternatively (if the consumption approach is being used), as various items are being used in food preparation. Moreover, individuals within families might be given such recorders in which to report meals and snacks purchased outside the home. The use of recorders could be especially useful in the case of less literate respondents.

DIARY CHECKING PROCEDURE

Some recent studies have indicated that there may be considerable disparities in the relative accuracy and completeness of reporting various food products in diaries. For example, comparatively costly items, such as meat and poultry, and perishable and frequently used products, such as milk, eggs, and bread, seem to be rather well reported, whereas food staples such as flour, sugar, and shortening tend to be seriously understated (Pearl, 1978). There appears to be a need, therefore, for special checking procedures to correct for these imbalances.

Some general checking procedures are specified in most diary operations, but what may be needed are specific sets of check questions aimed at those product categories most commonly underreported. In fact, the entire process may become much more of a combination of diaries and interviews than has usually been the case. A companion approach might be to take a brief shelf inventory of these types of staple products, at the time the diaries are being collected, and to inquire about the date of purchase of any that are found in order to determine whether the information was properly recorded.

WASTAGE

It is difficult to review the literature without finding a good deal of hand wringing about the inability to measure waste in food use (Pearl, 1977).

This writer has no inspired solutions to offer for this long-standing problem. Instead of the rather futile attempts to measure this element as part of a regular consumption survey, however, it might be more useful to carry out a series of small-scale studies devoted specifically to finding out how much of various food items are ordinarily wasted. Some spot visits to small household samples might be made right after the various meals to obtain quick information of this kind. Respondents might also be asked to record wastage on portable tape recorders, etc. In any event, the objective would be to develop adjustment factors that could be used to discount the usual purchase or consumption data prior to conversion to nutrients.

MEALS EATEN OUT

Another matter of some discouragement has been the impracticality of obtaining reliable information from survey respondents on the contents of meals eaten out. Since one out of every three food dollars is now spent in this manner, and the ratio is expected to rise to one in two, this problem is rather central in any effort to measure dietary adequacy. One possibility, in addition to obtaining whatever descriptions can be provided by respondents of meals eaten out, would be to record the names and addresses of the eating places. The objective (and this again might be attempted only for small samples) would be to solicit the recipes and lists of ingredients directly from the eating places (hopefully avoiding trade secrets). From a succession of such investigations, a glossary could possibly be developed that—at least in nutrient form—could describe a large proportion of meals eaten out (the preponderance of meals eaten in syndicated fast food establishments could help in this respect). Although obviously not without limitations, this approach could possibly improve what is one of the weakest links in the chain of dietary measurements.

INDICATOR FOODS

One of the problems in many complex surveys is that so vast an array of information is solicited that respondents experience memory failures or failures of execution, and survey personnel become so lost in the details that they are unable to institute adequate checking procedures. An apparent solution would be to reduce the amount of information to be requested from any one respondent, that is, in our immediate field of interest, to ask only about selected foods instead of the entire gamut. Since we are interested in the overall dietary adequacy of individual families and persons, the question is how to accomplish a reduction in detail without defeating the main objectives of the inquiry.

One possibility would be to attempt to develop a set of "indicator" foods, that is, a selection of foods that when translated into nutrient form would approximate the nutrient value of the complete diet of a given family or individual. This approach would represent a form of sampling similar to that used in estimating the overall price index from only a "market basket" of items. The data for the indicator foods would, of course, have to be appropriately weighted to arrive at a total nutrient value. In fact, regression equations might be developed to aid the estimation.

Various means might be utilized in the development of indicator lists. The knowledge and experience of dietary specialists would represent an important input. Experiments could be conducted with complete data sets (such as those from the ARS Food Consumption Surveys (see Murray, 1975), whereby various successive samples of items could be drawn and compared in nutrient value with the total consumption of the family or individual. For every item on an indicator list, there could be two or three options, in case the family did not use a particular product. Moreover, it would probably be necessary to develop different indicator lists for the various geographic regions, socioeconomic groups, and season of the year.

REFERENCES

Ferber, R., and S. Sudman. 1971. Experiments in obtaining consumer expenditure data by diary methods, J. Am. Stat. Assoc. 66:336, December.

Murray, J. 1975. Household food consumption surveys of the U.S. Department of Agriculture: A historical review of data collection methods, 1894–1969. Agricultural Research Service.

Pearl, R. B. 1977. Data systems on food demand and consumption: Properties, uses, future prospects. Pages 116–139 *in* Food demand and consumption behavior. Workshop sponsored by the S-119 Southern Regional Research Committee, State Agricultural Experiment Stations, and the Farm Foundation, Atlanta, March.

Pearl, R. B. 1978. The 1972–73 U.S. Consumer Expenditure Survey: A preliminary evaluation. U.S. Bureau of the Census Technical Paper Series. In press.

Quackenbush, G. G., and J. D. Shaffer. 1960. Collecting food purchase data by consumer panel. Mich. State Univ. Agric. Exp. Stn. Tech. Bull. 279. East Lansing, Mich.

Report and recommendations to the food and nutrition service on a proposed national food stamp program consumer panel survey. April 1976. Unpublished.

APPENDIX

C Background Papers for Workshop on Nutrition and Health Status Indicators

Can Nutritional Status Be Determined from Food Consumption or Other Measures?

A. E. SCHAEFER

I vividly recall the frustrations we had in developing and editing the *Manual for Nutrition Surveys* by the ICNND in 1957 followed by a second edition in 1963. In the early days of the ICNND's country nutrition surveys, there was immediate recognition of the need for a procedural manual that would:

1. Establish uniformity in methods, techniques, procedures, and guidelines for conducting surveys in population groups in order to make meaningful comparisons of results within and between countries. It was recognized that in some instances more refined and precise methods were known; however, for fieldwork as in population surveys, methods were selected that had the advantage of practicability, simplicity, and reproducibility. The interpretative guidelines for the biochemical data were developed for use of the methods cited.
2. Outline and define responsibilities of each segment of investigation (clinical examination, anthropometric, dietary, food production and processing).
3. Provide a guide for interpretation of the dietary, biochemical and clinical data.
4. Serve as a working reference of major facts essential for appraisal of nutritional status and to aid in interpretation of findings in order to draft practical recommendations to alleviate those nutritional problems discovered.
5. Assist in training personnel in nutrition appraisal techniques.

APPRAISAL METHODS

The general objectives of a nutrition survey are to define dietary intake at the time of the study; describe dietary patterns of consumption and food preparation practices; assess evidence concerning the prevalence of clinical, physical, biochemical, and anthropometric measurements indicative of nutritional status; and identify programs for improvement. This combined appraisal (dietary, biochemical, physical, anthropometric) gives more meaningful information than any single type of study. Biochemical studies provide means for estimating the proportion of the population in various broad zones of nutriture and provide an estimate of tissue reserves of the various nutrients. Dietary studies constitute an essential part of nutritional appraisal providing essential information for solution of problems uncovered. In a population survey, additional information should be collected, such as infant and child-feeding practices, school and institutional feeding, economy of food use, and the unique nutrient contribution of special foods.

Of the various methods of appraisal, biochemical and anthropometric measurements provide the key hard-core data, applicable to an individual or population group, for diagnosis of nutritional status and provide basic data to follow improvement or further deterioration. Dietary data is restricted in use; it does not define nutritional status. It is not a diagnostic measure. All of us appreciate the limitations of a 1-day, or 3-day, 7-day, or 30-day, etc., dietary assessment be it determined by recall or food weighings.

Of concern is the perpetual argument reference the validity and value of a 24-hour dietary recall versus the 1- to 3- to 7-day home record ± food weighings. Should we even waste time in doing it?

COMPARISON OF DIETARY INTAKE METHODS

Central America, INCAP–ICNND Survey

Dietary surveys in the six Central American countries included a comparison of the following methodology: In the case of families, food consumption was estimated by a 3-day daily record, a 24-hour recall with two different approaches (interviews in the home and interviews at the clinic), and a 1-day direct food weighing. For preschool children, a 1-day direct weighing and a 3-day daily record were used. The population sample for Nicaragua included a total of 125 families randomly divided in two groups. The 24-hour recall at home and the daily 3-day record were applied to the first group of families, while the 24-hour recall at the clinic and a 1-day direct weighing were applied to the second group of families (Table 1).

A comparison of the data obtained on the family studies revealed small differences that were not statistically significant. On the other hand, com-

TABLE 1 Comparison of Nutrient Intake by Different Methods in Families in Rural Nicaragua

		24-Hour Recall		3-Day Daily	1-Day Direct
		In Home	In Clinic	Record	Weighing
Calories	$\bar{x}$	1,928	1,857	1,916	1,950
	SD	702	639	683	674
Protein, g	$\bar{x}$	66.1	61.1	60.6	62.8
	SD	26.1	23.2	22.4	24.2
Calcium, mg	$\bar{x}$	725	790	773	755
	SD	455	572	457	438
Iron, mg	$\bar{x}$	17.8	16.6	18.7	17.9
	SD	8.1	7.7	7.9	10.5
Retinol, mcg	$\bar{x}$	150	98	169	247
	SD	569	86	570	1,270
Beta carotene, mcg	$\bar{x}$	522	481	578	527
	SD	591	525	630	642
Thiamin, mg	$\bar{x}$	0.87	0.82	0.92	0.91
	SD	0.38	0.30	0.40	0.42
Riboflavin, mg	$\bar{x}$	0.95	0.93	0.97	0.93
	SD	0.55	0.52	0.58	0.52
Niacin, mg	$\bar{x}$	10.90	9.89	10.26	9.97
	SD	5.28	3.47	4.01	3.74
Vitamin C, mg	$\bar{x}$	75	59	71	57
	SD	80	57	133	70

parison of the data of the preschool children revealed significant differences when comparing the 1-day direct weighing with the 3-day daily record for calcium, retinol, and riboflavin. For retinol and riboflavin, the differences were highly significant with the lower estimates found by the 1-day direct weighing (Table 2).

Examples of Use of Data—Central America Nutrition Surveys, 1965–67. In a study of over 3,800 families (approximately 20,000 people) in the six Central American countries, dietary intake studies were made on a sample of families on which detailed biochemical and hematological investigations were carried out. Two methods of obtaining quantitative data on family food consumption were used: one by means of a 24-hour recall, using the

TABLE 2 Comparison of Nutrient Intake by Various Methods in Preschool Children in Rural Nicaragua

		1-Day Direct Weighing	3-Day Daily Record
Calories	$\bar{x}$	1,089	1,100
	SD	< 142	433
Protein, g	$\bar{x}$	31.9	34.0
	SD	13.7	15.8
Calcium, mg	$\bar{x}$	413	693
	SD	294[a]	606[a]
Iron, mg	$\bar{x}$	9.0	8.1
	SD	6.0	4.0
Retinol, mcg	$\bar{x}$	47	130
	SD	49[b]	168[b]
Beta carotene	$\bar{x}$	167	300
	SD	171[a]	287[a]
Thiamin, mg	$\bar{x}$	0.44	0.50
	SD	0.24	0.21
Riboflavin, mg	$\bar{x}$	0.47	0.94
	SD	0.33[b]	0.80[b]
Vitamin C, mg	$\bar{x}$	28	32
	SD	36	33

[a] Significant at 5 percent probability.
[b] Significant at 1 percent probability.
NOTE: $\bar{x}$ = mean; SD = standard deviation.

housewife's own account of the previous day's meals; the other a 3-day record consisting of the actual recording in the home of the foods prepared and consumed. The 3-day record method was applied to a random portion of the families surveyed by the 24-hour recall.

At the end of the survey in each location, typical family diets were calculated and *food composites* were locally prepared for subsequent chemical analysis. Individual food intakes of preschool children were recorded by the 24-hour recall in most of the countries. The value and kinds of use of dietary data are illustrated in Tables 3–7.

The intake of vitamin A revealed a dramatic deficit when compared to the recommended levels of vitamin A. This finding was supported by the

TABLE 3 Consumption of Selected Foods per Person per Day in Rural Areas (g, Edible Portion)

Foods	Guatemala[a]	El Salvador	Honduras	Nicaragua	Costa Rica	Panama
Milk products[b]	84	190	194	243	193	73
Eggs	13	10	13	12	15	11
Meat, poultry, and fish	44	37	41	58	40	90
Beans and oily seeds	54	59	56	72	57	20
Vegetables	66	53	51	27	66	25
Fruits	14	17	40	41	7	50
Bananas and plantains	20	16	43	72	47	99
Starchy roots and tubers	14	13	22	33	46	82
Cereal products						
Rice	16	27	29	54	100	186
Corn tortillas, etc.[c]	359	352	224	139	41	32
Wheat bread	36	26	12	28	54	37
Wheat flour and pastes	4	0	8	7	12	10
Others	2	6	5	16	0	0
Sugar	52	41	39	58	89	51
Fats and oil	4	15	16	19	19	26
Number of families	203	293	331	355	456	361

[a]In the report on Guatemala (INCAP V-25), the figures for food consumption were those obtained by the 3-day-record method. In order to conform to the data in the reports for the other five countries, the dietary data for Guatemala used throughout this report are based on the 24-hour-recall method.

[b]In terms of liquid milk.

[c]In terms of grain.

TABLE 4 Percent Contribution of Selected Foods to Calorie Intake of Rural Families

Foods	Guatemala	El Salvador	Honduras	Nicaragua	Costa Rica	Panama
Milk products	2.8	5.6	6.9	7.3	7.3	2.7
Eggs	1.0	0.7	1.1	0.9	1.3	0.8
Meat, poultry, and fish	3.9	3.3	5.0	5.4	3.8	7.2
Beans and oily seeds	9.5	9.7	10.7	13.0	10.7	3.9
Vegetables	1.4	0.9	1.4	0.6	2.2	1.1
Fruits	0.6	0.6	1.8	1.5	0.4	4.1
Bananas and plantains	1.1	1.0	2.9	4.8	3.2	5.9
Starchy roots and tubers	0.6	0.7	1.8	2.2	2.6	4.9
Cereal products	65.1	61.8	49.5	41.5	39.3	47.4
Sugar	9.4	7.4	8.2	11.5	17.9	8.8
Fats and oil	2.6	6.9	8.8	9.3	9.8	11.7

TABLE 5 Average Intake of Calories and Specific Nutrients per Person per Day in Rural Families

	Guatemala	El Salvador	Honduras	Nicaragua	Costa Rica	Panama
Calories	2,117	2,146	1,832	1,986	1,894	2,089
Total protein, g	68.0	67.9	58.0	64.4	53.6	60.1
Animal protein, g	15.4	17.3	18.5	23.4	18.5	26.6
Vitamin A., IU	2,420	900	1,280	1,700	1,800	1,830
Riboflavin, mg	0.80	0.78	0.79	0.93	0.84	0.69
Iron, mg	17.9	11.6	15.5	18.2	15.4	14.3

TABLE 6 Percent Adequacy of Average Intake of Calories and Specific Nutrients in Rural Families

	Guatemala	El Salvador	Honduras	Nicaragua	Costa Rica	Panama
Calories	109	109	89	96	91	104
Protein	133	128	108	115	98	112
Vitamin A	68	24	34	44	49	49
Riboflavin	70	66	64	75	68	58
Iron	178	114	152	175	150	141

TABLE 7 Percent Distribution of Rural Families by Adequacy of Vitamin A Intake

Country	No. of Families	Percent Adequacy				
		<25	25–49	50–74	75–99	≥100
Guatemala	200	44	22	10	6	17
El Salvador	278	69	19	7	3	2
Honduras	323	57	26	9	2	6
Nicaragua	331	45	23	13	8	11
Costa Rica	414	44	26	11	7	12
Panama	352	42	32	13	5	8

biochemical evidence. Likewise when the data were analyzed by "low," "medium," and "high" socioeconomic index (Figure 1), the serum vitamin A concentration or urinary riboflavin values were lower in the poorer socioeconomic groups.

The incidence of clinical symptoms specifically related to nutrient deficiencies was not as high as the occurrence of biochemical values in the "deficient" or "high risk" range. This is to be expected.

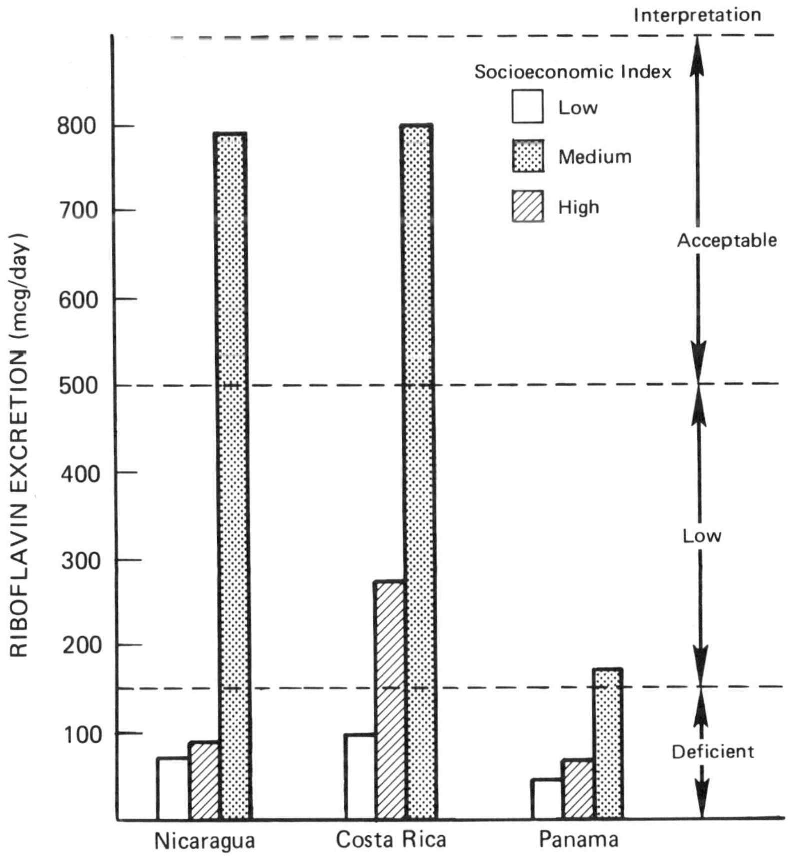

FIGURE 1 Nutritional study in Central America and Panama: Urinary excretion of riboflavin in relation to the socioeconomic index of the families in the rural areas of Central America, 1965–1967, males 0–4 yr.

Dietary studies revealed an even higher incidence of inadequate nutrient intakes than was evident from the biochemical and clinical studies.

The results of the biochemical analyses and dietary studies (with exception of vitamin A and riboflavin) indicated that the average consumption of essential nutrients in each country would have been enough if the distribution of the foods had been equitable.

Important differences in the average consumption of various foods per person per day was observed between countries. Likewise, these differences were observed between rural and urban families within each country. The basic dietary data correlated with biochemical estimates for those groups at "risk" or at "moderate risk" developing "malnutrition." No attempt to directly relate individual dietary intake to biochemical data *was done* nor should it *have been done*.

For defining the problems and potential solutions, it made no difference whatever which set of dietary intake data were used.

Bangladesh Nutrition Survey—Correlation of Diet and Biochemical Assessment

In the 1960–62 nutrition survey conducted in Bangladesh (then East Pakistan) (Pakistan, 1969), in which over 25,000 individuals were studied over a 2-year cycle, seasonal variations of intake of leafy green and yellow vegetables and fruits correlated with seasonal variations in serum vitamin A levels and the prevalence of keratomalacia. During the season when leafy green vegetables and yellow fruits were in short supply with an average daily consumption of only 12 g per day, 42 percent of the people had serum vitamin A levels of less than 20 mcg per 100 ml (Figure 2). Likewise, the percent of total cases seen at the Dacca medical college eye clinic with keratomalacia increases from 0.5 to 3.0 percent during the period of low intake of leafy green and yellow vegetables and fruits.

A similar type correlation was noted on the influence of pulse consumption on serum albumin levels (Figure 3). When intake reached a low level of 12 g of pulses per day, 58 percent of the population had "low" serum albumin levels of less than 3.5 g per 100 ml, whereas during periods of the year when pulse consumption reached 40 g per day, only 28 percent had "low" serum albumin levels.

Ecuador—ICNND Nutrition Survey

The Ecuador nutrition survey conducted in 1959 employed three methods of obtaining food consumption data: 24-hour recall, 24-hour recipe food weighing, and food composite chemical analysis. Comparisons of the nutrients consumed in two major regions (coastal and sierra) are given in Tables 8 and 9. The amounts of food consumed per person per day as determined by the direct recipe weighing method in the home and the 24-hour recall were in remarkably close agreement. The data illustrated that the results obtained from the recall questionnaire can be considered essentially as valid as the data obtained from direct weighings. The same number of personnel were required to obtain data from 28 families by the recipe weighing method as it took to obtain data from 341 families by the recall method. Food composites structured after the data obtained by the recipe method were analyzed by two laboratories.

The study revealed that in general the dietary recall method slightly un-

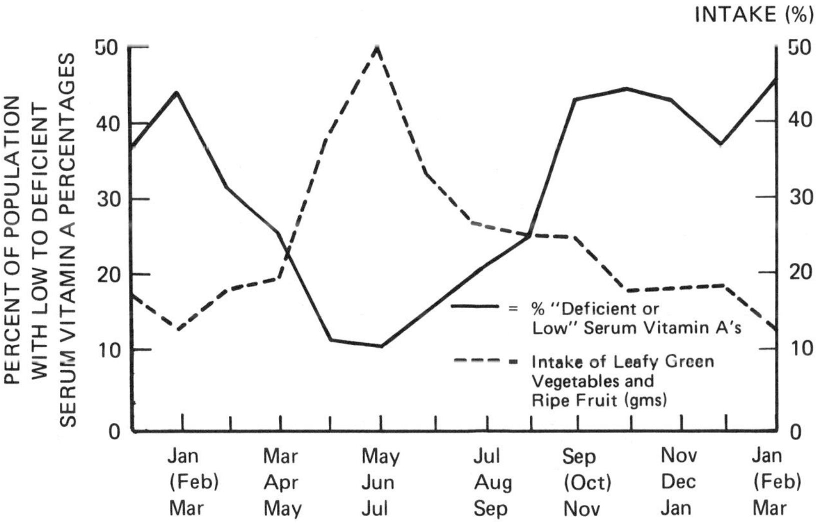

FIGURE 2 East Pakistan Nutrition Survey. Seasonal correlation of intake of leafy green vegetables and ripe fruit with serum vitamin A levels, 3-monthly averages.

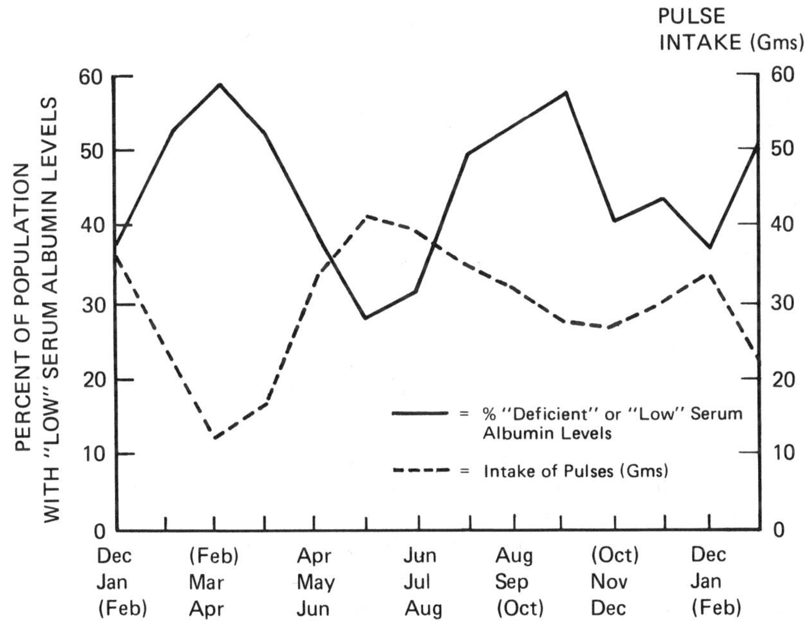

FIGURE 3 East Pakistan Nutrition Survey. Seasonal correlation of pulse intake with serum albumin levels, 3-monthly averages.

TABLE 8 ICNND Ecuador: Comparison of Average Daily Nutrient Intake (1959): Sierra Civilians

	NCR Calc. Allowance, 213 Families	24-Hour Recall, 213 Families	24-Hour Recipe Food Weigh, 15 Families	Food Composite Chemical, 15 Families
Calories	2,057	2,068	1,783	1,935
Protein, g	55	58	59	69
Calcium, g	1.04	0.49	0.47	0.61
Iron, mg	11.0	22.3	17.1	32.5
Vitamin A, IU	4,287	4,245	1,453	3,450
Thiamin, mg	1.18	1.17	1.0	0.82
Riboflavin, mg	1.64	0.81	0.91	1.68
Niacin, mg	16.0	22.2	20.8	20.3
Vitamin C, mg	71.0	112.0[a]	77.0[a]	54

[a]No cooking losses calculated.

TABLE 9 ICNND Ecuador: Comparison of Average Daily Nutrient Intake (1959): Coastal Civilians

	NCR Allowance, 116 Families	24-Hour Recall, 116 Families	24-Hour Recipe Food Weigh, 13 Families	Food Composite Chemical, 13 Families
Calories	1,878	1,791	1,769	1,940
Protein, g	53.3	58.2	57.2	63.3
Calcium, g	1.04	0.32	0.32	0.60
Iron, mg	11.0	14.0	14.1	21.0
Vitamin A, IU	4,042	4,554	3,524	2,614
Thiamin, mg	1.13	0.68[a]	0.68[a]	0.39
Riboflavin, mg	1.57	0.69	0.65	0.73
Niacin, mg	14.0	11.5	19.4	15.1
Vitamin C, mg	62.0	97.0[a]	86.0[a]	47

[a]No cooking losses calculated.

derestimates the food consumed by 10–15 percent. However, when larger numbers of families were studied, such as 341 families versus 28, the values for the recall method were equal or greater than the results obtained by the home recipe weighing method.

The food composite analysis method, which does require food intake data, provides the opportunity to obtain data on nutrient losses during cooking and on many nutrients for which food nutrient composition data were not available (vitamin B_6, folic acid, zinc, sodium, potassium, etc.). Chemical analyses of food composites in general include local water and local food preparation. In virtually all cases, higher iron and calcium values were found.

DIETARY METHODS IN EPIDEMIOLOGIC STUDIES

Morgan *et al.* (1978), as well as unpublished data by Margaret Moore and co-workers at Louisiana State University and Tulane, conclude that, ". . . Dietary history properly taken for research purposes serves a very useful purpose and is of greater value than is generally appreciated." Tests for reliability showed no significant differences in the values obtained within 2 years for a dietary history and 7-day food records. Morgan *et al.* employed three methods: 24-hour recall, 4-day dietary record, and diet history for 2 months, plus a recall for 2 months dating back 8 months. There was a high correlation between the current diet history intake and that measured 8 months previously. Current history data correlated with the 24-hour recall and the 4-day record. When all three methods were directed to the same period, they measured the same things. Although each method may be satisfactory for comparing group values, there is doubt as to which, if any, of the three methods is satisfactory for interpreting individual values. The authors concluded that the 24-hour recall and even the 4-day diary are inherently less reliable for individual estimates of usual intake and that when such estimates are required, the diet history should be used.

SUMMARY

The constraints of dietary survey are known by anyone familiar with human biology. Why one would expect a high degree of sensitivity is beyond comprehension. If one begins with crude data on nutrient composition, then why try to over interpret the data? For example, we continually see intense discussions and conclusions on precise intakes of fat, protein, carbohydrate, and fiber. The data in the data bank still represent carbohydrate values on the basis of "crude fiber determination" and in agricultural biochemistry terminology we talk about "proximate analysis." These are the first constraints of dietary intake data, unless one is willing to *really invest dollars* instead of talk in obtaining better than "proximate crude analysis data" to define such key nutrients as carbohydrates, fat, protein, crude fiber, and resultant calories.

On the positive side, one can interpret dietary intake data on population groups. An example of dietary intake correlating with biochemical assessment is illustrated by Figure 4.

From a practical slant, undoubtedly the most important findings relative to identifying diet patterns, habits, and food availability are data that define

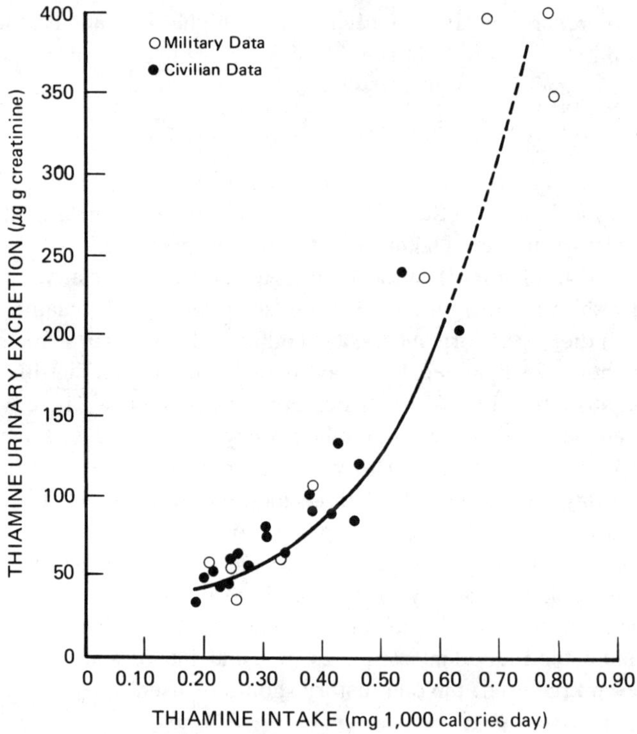

FIGURE 4 Relationship between thiamine intake and thiamine urinary excretion in adults of 18 countries. Data from civilian and military groups surveyed by the Interdepartmental Committee on Nutrition for National Defense of the United States of America. From: FAO Nutrition Meetings Report Series No. 41.

foods or food groups with estimates of quantitative intake. Note Table 10, which illustrates major variations in foods consumed between countries (Chile and Ecuador) and within regions of a country. For planning purposes from a health–economic–social standpoint, it is imperative to have such data on foods consumed.

TABLE 10 Representative Diet Patterns

	Chile	Ecuador (Lowlands)	Ecuador (Highlands)
Type of diet	wheat	rice	corn
No. of families	278	116	213
	g consumed per person per day		
Wheat products	351	35	39
Rice	23	122	79
Corn	—	2	116
Beef and mutton	81	66	42
Pork	9	—	—
Poultry	10	—	—
Fish	33	22	
Milk products	107	124	267
Eggs	8	8	2
Fats and oils	27	38	11
Leafy green and yellow vegetables	97	57	38
Potatoes	153	125	275
Tomatoes	16	30	6
Other vegetables	46	20	21
Pulses	27	20	39
Citrus fruit	5	21	13
Bananas	6	99	19
Other	96	—	

[a] ICNND Survey Reports—1960, Chile; 1959, Ecuador.

REFERENCES AND BIBLIOGRAPHY

Archivos Latino Americanos de Nutricion, Vol. XXIII, Sept. 1973, pp. 325–344. Marina Flores, María Teresa Menchú, and Miguel A. Guzmán. Evalución dietética de familias y preescolares mediante la aplicación de diferentes métodos y tecnicas—Area rural de Nicaragua.

Ecuador. Nutrition Survey, 1959. Report by the ICNND, July 1960. Published by NIAMD, HEW, Bethesda, Md.

Manual for Nutrition Surveys, 2d ed. 1963. Interdepartmental Committee on Nutrition for National Defense, National Institutes of Health, Bethesda, Md. U.S. Government Printing Office, Washington, D.C.

Morgan, R. W., *et al.*, 1978. A comparison of dietary methods in epidemiologic studies. Am. J. Epidemiol., 107(6):488–498.

Pakistan. Nutrition Survey, March 1962–January 1964. 1969. Report by the Ministry of Health, Gov't. Pakistan, University of Dacca. Nutrition Section of NIH, Department of HEW.

Relating Food Intake, Demographic, Attitudes and Behavior Data to Measures of Nutritional Status

HOWARD G. SCHUTZ

Other than for major deficiencies in intake, the relationship between dietary intake and health status has not been clearly delineated. Certainly for the objectives of the FDA, there is not available any generally accepted method for determining the possible relationships between consumption of food ingredients and health status.

There are three major problem areas associated with this task. First are the myriad of difficulties associated with the collection of reliable and valid data concerning individual food intake patterns. These difficulties have been discussed in a previous workshop. Second are the problems associated with the collection of meaningful measures of health status. These will be discussed at the present workshop. Among the questions to be answered are: (1) What is the value of self-reported health status? (2) What kind of biochemical data should be collected and for what period of time? (3) What nonbiochemical attitude behavior and demographic measures are appropriate to collect? Third is the problem of how we relate our measures of food intake and other variables to the health status measures.

The latter issue is the one that I would like to address. I believe the assumption that relationships can and should be studied between single measures of intake and nonintake and health status is simplistic. There is every reason to believe that there are additive and perhaps interactive effects among nutrients that contribute to particular health conditions. Also, it is quite likely that measures of attitude and behavior, as well as demographic characteristics, can play an important role alone and in combination with intake to influence health measures.

What appears to me to be one approach to the problem of determining relationships is to relate measures of intake and other variables to health status utilizing a multivariate approach. Using the statistical method of multiple regression, the intake, demographic, attitude, and behavior variables become the independent variables and the particular measure of health status becomes the dependent variable. This approach in its simplest form yields the linear additive relationships between the predictor variables, i.e., intake, etc., and the dependent variables, a health status measure. By utilizing squared and cross-multiplied terms, one can also include nonlinear effects and interactions.

As an aid in reducing and simplifying the independent and sometimes the dependent variable, I have used a clustering technique such as factor analysis first in order to select variables that represent fundamental dimensions and that are not related to one another statistically.

Four examples of the general approach are noted. The first of three papers (Schutz *et al.*, 1977) is a paper on predicting purchase and use that does not measure health status but does demonstrate the multivariate approach to the general areas of food. The second (Baird and Schutz, 1976) is a paper that demonstrates the approach applied to predicting judged dietary adequacy for four ethnic groups using cognitive structure based on food-appropriateness information as independent variables. The third paper (Baird and Schutz, 1980) demonstrates the successful prediction of a number of measures of nutritional status by demographic and attitudinal variables. These data were for a sample of 100 Californians.

The fourth example consists of summary tables showing the results of a multivariate analysis of intake, demographic attitude and behavior, and nutritional status data collected (*N* varies from 349 to 435) on female heads of households in five Western states. These data are from an experiment station bulletin that is in press. Table 1 gives the variables studied and Tables 2–11 give stepwise multiple regression results for nine measures of health status. Three regressions are given, one with only environmental variables (demographic I), one with environmental plus attitude and behavior variables (IIa), and the third with environmental, attitude, and behavior, plus dietary intake (III). Examination of the tables reveals that statistically significant predictions were possible in all cases but that the variance accounted for varied from about 1 percent to 70 percent. I view the results in this last set of tables as very encouraging, since measures of intake were only 3-day diet records, biochemical measures were single occasion measures, and most importantly five different sets of experimenters collected the data. More reliable and valid data collection techniques should result in the ability to predict higher amounts of variance in the health status variables.

REFERENCES

Baird, P. C., and H. G. Schutz. 1976. The marketing concept applied to "selling" good nutrition. J. Nutr. Educ. 8:13–17.

Baird, P. C., and H. G. Schutz. 1980. Dietary and nutritional status: Life style correlates. J. Am. Diet. Assoc. 76:228–235.

Schutz, H. G., S. M. Moore, and M. H. Ricker. 1977. Predicting food purchase and use by multivariate attitudinal analysis. Food Tech. 31:85–92.

(See tables overleaf and following pages)

TABLE 1 List of Variables. (*Indicates Dummy Variable, 1 = Yes, 0 = No)

1. NUTRITIONAL STATUS MEASURES
   a. *Anthropometric and Clinical Measures* (dependent variables, regressions I, IIa, III)
      1. Triceps skinfold thickness, mm
      2. Diastolic blood pressure, mm Hg
   b. *Biochemical Measures* (dependent variables, regressions I, IIa, III)
      3. Total serum protein, g/dl
      4. Iron binding capacity, μg/dl
      5. Serum albumin, g/dl
      6. Plasma vitamin A, μg/dl
      7. Serum iron, μg/dl
      8. Hematocrit, %
      9. Serum vitamin C, mg/dl
      10. Iron transferrin saturation, %
   c. *Dietary Intake* (mean intake from food and supplements/day) (dependent variables, regressions I, IIa; independent variables, regression III)
      11. Carbohydrate intake, g
      12. Viamin C intake, mg
      13. Niacin intake, mg
      14. Vitamin A intake, IU
      15. Protein intake, g
      16. Thiamin intake, mg
      17. Riboflavin intake, mg
      18. Iron intake, mg
      19. Energy intake, kcal
      20. Calcium intake, mg
      21. Phosphorus intake, mg
      22. Fat intake, g

2. FOOD ACCEPTANCE MEASURES (dependent variables, regressions I, IIb; independent variables, regression IIa)
      23. Frequency scale (freq scale)—average frequency of serving 174 foods (high scores = low frequency)
      24. Like–dislike scale (like/dislike)
      25. "Finicky" scale (finicky)
      26. Vitamin usage—number of vitamin pills taken daily (vit pill user)

3. ENVIRONMENTAL FACTORS (independent variables)
   a. *Selected Physical, Socioeconomic, and Social Environmental Factors* (selected before the study commenced) (regressions I, IIa&b, III)
      27. Age (yr), varies from (18–57 yr)
      *28. Ethnic group—(nonwhite) (reference = caucasian)
      29. Income—annual family income (income)
         1. Less than $3,000
         2. 3,000–5,999
         3. 6,000–8,999
         4. 9,000–11,999
         5. 12,000–24,999
         6. Over 25,000

TABLE 1 *Continued*

30. Number of persons living in household (# persons), including the respondent (varies from 1–over 11) (household size)
31. Highest level of education completed by (educ) lead female
    1. 5 grades or less
    2. 6–8 grades
    3. 9–11 grades
    4. High school graduate
    5. Some technical training or college
    6. Junior/community college graduate
    7. College graduate
    8. Graduate school
32. Rural/urban—size of community
    1. Small rural community, <1,000 people
    2. Rural community, 1,000–2,500
    3. Small community, 2,500–10,000
    4. Small urban community, 10,000–25,000
    5. Large urban community, 25,000–50,000
    6. Metropolis, 50,000 and over

*33. State—Arizona
*34. State—Hawaii
*35. State—Nevada
*36. State—Washington
} Reference = California

b. *Other Factors Hypothesized to Affect Nutritional Status and/or Food Acceptance* (independent variables, regressions IIa, b, III)

i. *Activity factors*

*37. Employed (yes = 1, no = 0)

38. Job activity level
    1. Sedentary
    2. Mildly active
    3. Very active
39. DPAS = daily physical activity score. Total average hourly kilocaloric expenditures for each physical activity (swimming, exercising, walking, dancing, bowling, tennis, other specific listed by subject. If none, score was average hourly energy expenditure for sedentary office work.

ii. *Reasons for serving food to the family*. Number of times respondants mentioned reasons that fall into the following categories.

	Code
40. Sensory reason	1
41. Social reason	2
42. Education reason	3
43. Psychological reason	4
44. Emotional reason	5
45. Religious reason	6
46. Health reason	7
47. Preparation reason	9
48. Miscellaneous reason	10
49. Price reason	8.01, 8.02, 8.11
50. Availability reason	8.03, 8.08, 8.09

TABLE 1 *Continued*

51. "Do (grow/hunt) yourself" reason — 8.06, 8.08, 8.10

iii. *Consumer behavior factors*

*52. Don't buy any food more frequently than others (don't buy)
*53. Have no regular pattern of shopping for groceries (no reg shop)
*54. Shop on the weekends (shop w/e)
*55. Shop in chain supermarket (shop supermarket)
*56. Shop where get the lowest price (shop low price)
*57. Shop for maximum quality at minimum price (shop min/max)
*58. Not eligible for food stamps (ineligible FS)
*59. Would buy more meat if had more money (more meat)
*60. Would buy fewer sweets and snacks if had less money (fewer sweets/snacks)
*61. Have adequate kitchen storage (storage OK)
*62. Get food information from newspapers and magazines (info pop press)
*63. Shop when convenient (shop convenience)
*64. Has family members on special diet (special diet)

TABLE 2 Anthropometric and Clinical Measures—Triceps Skinfold Thickness, mm; Variable 1; Mean = 23.8 ± 8.1 (441)

Independent Variables			Regression I			Regression IIa			Regression III		
No.	Name	Correlation Coefficient	Slope Coeff.	Standz Slope Coeff.	Rank	Slope Coeff.	Standz Slope Coeff.	Rank	Slope Coeff.	Standz Slope Coeff.	Rank
		r	B	B*		B	B*		B	B*	
34	Hawaii	−0.140	−3.128	−0.145	1						
31	Education	−0.110	−0.742	−0.134	2	−0.603	−0.109	4	−0.625	−0.118	6
27	Age	+0.139	+0.117	+0.125	3	+0.129	+0.138	3	+0.125	+0.134	4
36	Washington	−0.079	−2.351	−0.124	4						
35	Nevada	+0.195	+2.391	+0.118	5	+3.015	+0.149	2	+2.704	+0.134	4
40	Sensory reason	+0.176				+0.055	+0.169	1	+0.048	+0.149	3
15	Protein intake	+0.071							+0.056	+0.162	1
11	CHO intake	−0.168							−0.168	−0.018	2
Number of independent variables included			10			42			64		
Constant (C)			23.614			19.607			19.061		
Mean square of regression (R)			0.292			0.300			0.361		
F value of Regression (F)			7.40[a]			9.04[a]			7.76[a]		
Percent of variation explained (%)			8.6			9.0			13.0		

[a] Significant at $p < 0.01$.

TABLE 3 Anthropometric and Clinical Measures—Diastolic Blood Pressure, mm Hg; Variable 2; Mean = 78 ± 41 (381)

Independent Variables			Regression I			Regression IIa			Regression III		
No.	Name	Correlation Coefficient	Slope Coeff.	Standz Slope Coeff.	Rank	Slope Coeff.	Standz Slope Coeff.	Rank	Slope Coeff.	Standz Slope Coeff.	Rank
		r	B	B*		B	B*		B	B*	
27	Age	+0.108	+0.516	+0.108	1	+0.492	+0.103	3	+0.522	+0.110	7
38	Job activity	+0.113				+7.342	+0.170	1	+7.988	+0.186	4
37	Employed	−0.052				−5.930	−0.124	2	−6.273	−0.131	6
16	Thiamin intake	+0.219							+4.216	+0.784	1
17	Riboflavin intake	+0.105							−1.945	−0.328	2
13	Niacin intake	+0.029							−0.334	−0.298	3
20	Calcium intake	−0.047							−0.010	−0.143	5
57	Shop max/min	+0.096							+10.765	+0.100	8
Number of independent variables included			10			42			64		
Constant (C)			57.857			51.200			57.475		
Mean square of regression (R)			0.108			0.192			0.420		
F value of regression (F)			4.367[a]			4.673[a]			10.198[a]		
Percent of variation explained (%)			1.2			3.7			18.4		

[a]Significant at $p < 0.05$.

TABLE 4 Biochemical Measures—Serum Total Protein, g/dl; Variable 3; Mean = 7.00 ± 0.63 (435)

Independent Variables			Regression I			Regression IIa			Regression III		
No.	Name	Correlation Coefficient	Slope Coeff.	Standz Slope Coeff.	Rank	Slope Coeff.	Standz Slope Coeff.	Rank	Slope Coeff.	Standz Slope Coeff.	Rank
		r	B	B*		B	B*		B	B*	
32	Rural/urban	+0.205	+0.201	+0.559	1	+0.631	+1.754	4	+0.631	1.754	4
34	Hawaii	−0.086	−0.866	−0.515	2	−5.929	−3.530	1	−5.930	−3.530	1
33	Arizona	−0.027	−0.703	−0.435	3	−3.839	−2.376	2	−3.839	−2.376	2
35	Nevada	−0.097	−0.592	−0.374	4	−1.580	−0.999	5	−1.580	−0.999	5
28	Ethnic nonwhite	+0.054	+0.166	+0.112	5	+0.750	+0.504	11	+0.750	+0.504	11
40	Sensory reason					−0.046	−1.835	3	−0.046	−1.835	3
36	Washington	−0.158				−2.325	−1.567	6	−2.325	−1.567	6
46	Health reason	+0.051				−0.040	−0.973	7	−0.040	−0.973	7
47	Preparation reason	−0.005				−0.043	−0.803	8	−0.043	−0.803	8

38	Job Activity	+0.037		+0.379	+0.577	9	+0.379	+0.577	9
23	Freq scale	−0.124		+0.350	+0.516	10	+1.421	+0.516	10
37	Employed	−0.034		+0.350	+0.479	12	+0.350	+0.479	12
49	Price reason	−0.008		−0.054	−0.463	13	−0.054	−0.463	13
50	Avail reason	−0.171		−0.082	−0.454	14	−0.082	−0.454	14
41	Social reason	−0.074		−0.022	−0.165	15	−0.022	−0.165	15
45	Religious	−0.195		−0.022	−0.094	16	−0.022	−0.094	16
Number of independent variables included			10	42			64		
Constant (C)			6.400	4.064			4.064		
Mean square of regression (R)			0.462	0.840			0.84		
F value of regression (F)			19.76[a]	52.69[a]			52.69		
Percent of variation explained (%)			21.3	70.5			70.5		

[a] Significant at $p < 0.001$.

TABLE 5 Biochemical Measures—Iron Binding Capacity (IBC) μg/dl; Variable 4; Mean = 348 ± 117 (371)

Independent Variables			Regression I			Regression IIa			Regression III		
No.	Name	Correlation Coefficient	Slope Coeff.	Standz Slope Coeff.	Rank	Slope Coeff.	Standz Slope Coeff.	Rank	Slope Coeff.	Standz Slope Coeff.	Rank
		r	B	B*	B	B*	B	B*			
32	Rural/urban	−0.355	− 67.262	−1.008	1	− 63.437	−0.954	1	− 68.437	−1.025	1
36	Washington	+0.164	−197.91	−0.719	2	−240.515	−0.973	2	−276.932	−1.006	2
34	Hawaii	−0.345	− 69.852	−0.224	3	−134.340	−0.431	3	−162.785	−0.522	3
35	Nevada	+0.294	+ 57.053	+0.194	4	+ 55.284	+0.188	5	+ 69.889	+0.238	5
28	Ethnic nonwhite	−0.087	+ 48.512	+0.176	5	+ 66.388	+0.240	4	+ 78.497	+0.284	4
23	Freq. scale	+0.061				+ 83.161	+0.163	6	+ 91.051	+0.178	7
40	Sensory reason	+0.102				− 0.725	−0.155	7	− 0.882	−0.189	6
41	Social reason	−0.107				− 3.324	−0.137	8	− 3.490	−0.144	8
61	Storage OK	−0.106				− 25.636	−0.100	9	− 25.533	−0.100	12

64	Special diet	−0.128				+ 22.321	+0.082	10	+ 27.603	+0.101	11
11	CHO intake	−0.006							+ 0.222	+0.138	9
45	Religious reason	+0.052							− 4.542	−0.106	10
46	Health reason	+0.111							− 0.711	−0.093	13
18	Iron intake	−0.061							− 0.312	−0.086	14
62	Info pop press	+0.016							− 22.635	−0.079	15
Number of independent variables included			10			42			64		
Constant (C)			705.84			473.44			473.529		
Mean square of regression (R)			0.599			0.639			0.665		
F value of regression (F)			40.75[a]			24.784[a]			18.704[a]		
Percent of variation explained (%)			35.9			40.8			44.2		

[a] Significant at $p < 0.001$.

TABLE 6 Biochemical Measures—Serum Albumin, g/dl; variable 5; Mean = 4.15 ± 0.40 (349)

Independent Variables			Regression I			Regression IIa			Regression III		
No.	Name	Correlation Coefficient	Slope Coeff.	Standz Slope Coeff.	Rank	Slope Coeff.	Standz Slope Coeff.	Rank	Slope Coeff.	Standz Slope Coeff.	Rank
		r	B	B*		B	B*		B	B*	
34	Hawaii	−0.509	−0.551	−0.514	1	−0.655	−0.612	1	−0.662	−0.618	1
27	Age	+0.059	−0.004	−0.088							
24	Like/dislike	+0.097				−0.921	−0.184	2	−0.932	−0.186	2
45	Religious reason	+0.014				−0.020	−0.132	3	−0.020	−0.139	3
38	DPAS	+0.186				+0.008	+0.098	4	+0.008	+0.105	4
30	Household size	+0.018				+0.013	+0.092	5	+0.014	+0.095	5
18	Iron intake	−0.041							−0.001	−0.920	6
Number of independent variables included			10			42			64		
Constant (C)			4.401			5.031			5.059		
Mean square of regression (R)			0.517			0.558			0.566		
F value of regression (F)			66.873[a]			32.953[a]			28.457		
Percent of variation explained (%)			26.7			31.2			32.0		

[a] Significant at $p < 0.001$.

TABLE 7 Biochemical Measures—Plasma Vitamin A, $\mu g/dl$; Variable 6; Mean = 79.5 ± 49.0 (414)

Independent Variables			Regression I			Regression IIa			Regression III		
No.	Name	Correlation Coefficient	Slope Coeff.	Standz Slope Coeff.	Rank	Slope Coeff.	Standz Slope Coeff.	Rank	Slope Coeff.	Standz Slope Coeff.	Rank
		r	B	B*		B	B*		B	B*	
35	Nevada	+0.219	+30.285	+0.247	1	+30.285	−0.247	1	+30.285	+0.247	1
33	Arizona	+0.246	+28.606	+0.228	2	+28.606	+0.228	2	+28.606	+0.228	2
32	Rural/urban	+0.326	+ 5.863	+0.210	3	+ 5.863	+0.210	3	+ 5.863	+0.210	3
Number of independent variables included			10			42			64		
Constant (C)			40.093			40.093			40.093		
Mean square of regression (R)			0.449			0.423			0.423		
F value of regression (F)			23.069[a]			26.563[a]			26.562[a]		
Percent of variation explained (%)			20.2			17.9			17.9		

[a]Significant at $p < 0.001$.

TABLE 8 Biochemical Measures—Serum Iron, μg/dl; Variable 7; Mean = 87.5 ± 39.1 (429)

Independent Variables			Regression I			Regression IIa			Regression III		
No.	Name	Correlation Coefficient	Slope Coeff.	Standz Slope Coeff.	Rank	Slope Coeff.	Standz Slope Coeff.	Rank	Slope Coeff.	Standz Slope Coeff.	Rank
		r	B	B*		B	B*		B	B*	
36	Washington	+0.242	+19.506	+0.212	1	+10.861	+0.118	4	+20.236	+0.220	2
34	Hawaii	−0.234	−18.163	−0.175	2	−30.657	−0.305	1	−23.362	−0.225	1
31	Education	+0.080	+ 2.650	+0.100	3	+ 2.931	+0.110	6			
26	Vit pill user	+0.076				+ 6.411	+0.143	2	+ 7.973	+0.178	3
46	Health reason	−0.097				− 0.360	−0.142	3			
49	Price reason	−0.056				−0.799	−0.111	5			
14	Vit A intake	−0.036							−0.000	−0.126	4
38	Job activity	−0.057							− 3.795	−0.093	5
Number of independent variables included			10			42			64		
Constant (C)			72.908			83.797			89.675		
Mean square of regression (R)			0.316			0.381			0.360		
F value of regression (F)			13.558[a]			8.791[b]			10.81[b]		
Percent of variation explained (%)			10.0			14.5			12.9		

[a] Significant at $p < 0.001$.
[b] Significant at $p < 0.01$.

TABLE 9 Biochemical Measures—Hematocrit, %; Variable 8; Mean = 41.2 ± 3.0 (350)

Independent Variables			Regression I			Regression IIa			Regression III		
No.	Name	Correlation Coefficient	Slope Coeff.	Standz Slope Coeff.	Rank	Slope Coeff.	Standz Slope Coeff.	Rank	Slope Coeff.	Standz Slope Coeff	Rank
		r	B	B*		B	B*		B	B*	
28	Ethnic nonwhite	−0.101	−1.063	−0.152	1	−0.826	−0.118	4	−0.756	−0.108	7
31	Education	−0.123	−0.279	−0.138	2	−0.261	−0.129	3	−0.268	−0.133	4
33	Arizona	−0.130	−0.972	−0.128	3						
29	Income	−0.109	−0.284	−0.112	4						
45	Religious reason	−0.160				−0.183	−0.168	1	−0.177	−0.162	1
48	Misc. reason	+0.174				+0.059	+0.154	2	+0.059	+0.155	2
15	Protein intake	−0.081							+0.018	+0.141	3
11	CHO Intake	−0.091							−0.005	−0.124	5
14	Vita A intake	−0.095							−0.000	−0.111	6
Number of independent variables included			10			42			64		
Constant (C)			44.216			42.362			42.264		
Mean square of regression (R)			0.247			0.286			0.336		
F value of regression (F)			5.947[a]			8.103[b]			6.6[a]		
Percent of variation explained (%)			6.1			8.2			11.3		

[a] Significant at $p < 0.05$.
[b] Significant at $p < 0.001$.

TABLE 10 Biochemical Measures—Serum Vitamin C, mg/dl; Variable 9; Mean = 1.31 ± 0.54 (419)

Independent Variables			Regression I			Regression IIa			Regression III		
No.	Name	Correlation Coefficient	Slope Coeff.	Standz Slope Coeff.	Rank	Slope Coeff.	Standz Slope Coeff.	Rank	Slope Coeff.	Standz Slope Coeff.	Rank
		r	B	B*		B	B*		B	B*	
32	Rural/urban	+0.168	0.060	0.191	1				+0.059	+0.191	2
28	Ethnic nonwhite	−0.046	0.128	0.101	2						
41	Social reason	+0.190				+0.018	+0.163	1			
46	Health reason	+0.144				+0.005	+0.140	2			
26	Vit pill user	+0.151				+0.079	+0.128	3			
37	Employed	−0.053				−0.064	−0.103	4			
39	DPAS	−0.083				−0.010	−0.093	5			
12	Vit C intake	+0.259							+0.001	+0.271	1
56	Shop low price								+0.134	+0.116	3
Number of independent variables included			10			42			64		
Constant (C)			1.050			1.202			0.883		
Mean square of regression (R)			0.194			0.289			0.335		
F value of regression (F)			7.175[a]			6.658[a]			15.382[b]		
Percent of variation explained (%)			3.8			8.4			11.2		

[a]Significant at $p < 0.01$.
[b]Significant at $p < 0.001$.

TABLE 11 Biochemical Variables—Iron Transferrin Saturation, %; Variable 10; Mean = 27.2 ± 13.6 (370)

Independent Variables			Regression I			Regression IIa			Regression III		
No.	Name	Correlation Coefficient	Slope Coeff.	Standz Slope Coeff.	Rank	Slope Coeff.	Standz Slope Coeff.	Rank	Slope Coeff.	Standz Slope Coeff.	Rank
		r	B	B*		B	B*		B	B*	
28	Ethnic	−0.187	−5.978	−0.187	1	−6.266	−0.196	1	−6.702	−0.210	1
26	Vit pill user	+0.098				+1.766	+0.114	2	+1.862	+0.120	2
21	Phosphorus intake	−0.066							−0.003	−0.100	3
Number of independent variables included			10			42			64		
Constant (C)			28.599			26.922			29.828		
Mean Square of regression (R)			0.187			0.219			0.240		
F value of regression (F)			13.342[a]			9.220[b]			7.461[b]		
Percent of variation explained (%)			3.5			4.8			5.8		

[a]Significant at $p < 0.001$
[b]Significant at $p < 0.01$.

Methods of Relating Food Consumption to Nutritional Status and Health: Dietary Methodology

VICTOR M. HAWTHORNE

SUMMARY

New national intiatives in promoting health and preventing disease in nutrition suggest need for awareness of the limitations of dietary methodology and its use in epidemiological studies designed to assess efficiency and effectiveness, determine "normal" values, compare rates, validate techniques and decide priorities.

Use of the four main quantitative methods of collecting dietary data are reviewed in relation to their use in cardiovascular disease, cancer, diabetes and obesity.

It is concluded that in epidemiological studies of nutrition, reliance can be placed on a combination of estimated current record, 24-hour recall and diet history adapted in frequency and extent to meet the design needs of individual studies. Quantitative assessments can be improved by use of new specifically designed food tables to derive nutrient values; and qualitative data collected from food frequency studies through a scoring system restricted to specific foods.

The need is postulated for a nutritional health information system incorporating facilities for medical record linkage allowing outcomes to be assessed against baseline values.

INTRODUCTION

Nutrition is the sum of the processes by which man uses natural and artificial substances ingested for the growth, maintenance, and repair of vital processes. Nutrition is related to metabolism, in itself the sum of all processes concerned with the anabolism and catabolism of protoplasm. Food, and more generally diet, cannot be considered in isolation from nutrition, which is the ultimate expression, for better or for worse, of what has or has not been taken into the body.

The aims of this review are to examine some adquacies and deficiencies in the use of dietary data as a means of assessing the extent to which nutrition is a determinant of cardiovascular disease, cancer, and allied chronic conditions; and to appraise at present the best use of these methods to monitor the effects of nutritional change on human health.

Epidemiologically the spectrum of nutrition corresponds to health and disease. Modified by heredity and subject to environment, nutrition depends on the same demographic factors. Studies must therefore be population-based and encompass optimal and suboptimal as well as frank, malnutritional states. Indeed, as in mild hypertension, intervention in suboptimal nutrition may offer the best interventive strategy. Epidemiology uses whole populations as denominators to provide the statistical basis for determining "normal" values, to compare rates in different populations, to validate diagnostic techniques, to implement field trials, to decide management priorities, and to coordinate the provision of appropriate, multidisciplinary skills in medicine, biochemistry, anthropology, physiology, sociology, demography, and biostatistics.

GENERAL METHODS

Literature purporting to describe the relationship between food intake patterns and chronic disease is as extensive as it is inconclusive, but describes a number of techniques common to the acquisition and use of dietary data.

Dietary intakes of households and individuals have been measured since 1900, but studies designed to relate diet and nutrition to health and disease were uncommon until the 1930's. Burk and Pao's review (1976) of the methodology for large-scale surveys of household and individual diets critically evaluates the four main quantitative methods of collecting data: the weighed record, the estimated record, 24-hour recall, and dietary history. Employing an extensive range of validating criteria, they conclude that no one method was consistently advantageous over all others and no selection could be made independently of study objectives.

Marr (1973) comments that, although details of weights or standard measures of food can be recorded at the time food is eaten, the demand on the participants adversely affects response. Recall makes least demand, but has the disadvantage of placing too great reliance on memory. Current record methods, on the other hand, avoid inaccuracies due to memory, but the study procedure itself may influence eating habits.

Both recall and record methods collect details of foods eaten, and tables of food composition must be used to derive nutrient values. The basis for calculation of these tables is suspect due to variation in conditions affecting growth and processing of food not provided for in the tables, a deficiency that can be overcome when comparing groups by using only the extremes of the distributions. Selective response in certain age and socioeconomic groups are another source of bias for which provision must be made. Day-to-day and week-to-week variation of diet affect the precision of most methods and influence considerations establishing the shortest period over which recall cán be used to estimate dietary intake. The greater within-person and day-to-day variation, compared with between-person variation, the longer should be the period of dietary recording. The type of nutrient introduces a further element of variation.

The measurement of nutritional status is in effect a measure of outcome. Dietary data must be combined with biochemical and clinical measurements with all their implications for cost in response and resources. As a general guide food intake can be used as a valid index of daily energy expenditure, but estimates must extend over a minimum period of a week.

CARDIOVASCULAR METHOD

The relationship of diet to cardiovascular disease was reviewed by Rose and Blackburn (1968) in the late 1960's. Like others, they fail to identify any single approach to assessing dietary intake but list the main methods in common use for epidemiological studies of ischemic heart disease. These again include direct measurement of food intake in which all food eaten by an individual or family is weighed or measured by a dietician in the home. This method is limited by time and cost. Results may not reflect seasonal variation and may be biased by the investigative process. The same reservations apply to the chemical analysis of food intake by collection of an approximate aliquot of each dish or food eaten.

Twenty-four-hour recall is described as simple, direct, and inexpensive. A tendency to underestimate intake may be remedied by adjusting the number of days covered to meet the objectives of the study.

Food diaries over 1 week with entries made at mealtimes and interviewer review either with or without weighing had already been adapted for postal use (Keen and Rose, 1958). Response problems, however, restricted use to literate populations.

Dietary history can be recorded on questionnaires (Burke, 1947) using a method incorporating cross-checks and with 24-hour recall as a further check. Apart from being time-consuming and expensive in staff and resources, the method needs careful work-up. Only usual diet is measured, past changes are excluded and much depends on the ability of the participant to define and recall usual food intake.

Abbreviated methods of collecting dietary data cheaply in epidemiological studies had not been attempted in the sixties, but have now been assessed (Hankin, 1978).

Instead of quantitating nutrient intake, frequency of intake of specified food can be used to develop a scoring system. This method has been used with 24-hour recall in the Tecumseh Population Study (Metzner *et al.*, 1977; Nichols *et al.*, 1976a,b).

Epidemiological studies have been used to arrive at mean values for population groups using these methods and to study the effects of dietary intervention on biological indices such as cholesterol. In these studies diet has to be assessed over the course of a year using statistical models like those of Becker and his colleagues (Becker *et al.*, 1960), who studied food intake in a time series approach. No satisfactory method of measuring long-term diet retrospectively has yet been established, and long-term prospective designs with interval sampling are recommended.

In assessing nutrients of special interests to cardiovascular disease, standard food table procedures have been inadequate. New chemical analyses now being made for food tables in respect of special terms of nutrients may enhance the value of food tables in future studies.

Rose and Blackburn (1968) comment on the relation of data collection to computer processing. They list the staging of data collection from tabulation of the quantity of food eaten in multiples of a predetermined unit of volume or weight dependent on the food tables to be used; reporting of food intake for a predetermined period; grouping of foods into combinations of similar nutritive value, perhaps using abbreviated food tables for this purpose; and the recording of other variables such as number of meals per day and meals away from home. As already mentioned, where nutrition is to be included as a form of outcome the data must be associated with biochemical, clinical, psychological, and sociological variables. Computer programs were already available from the Heart Disease Control Program of the U.S. Public Health Service and the Coronary Prevention Evaluation Program.

The role of diet and various dietary factors in ischemic heart disease has been reviewed recently by a working group on ischemic heart disease of the Chief Scientist Office of the Scottish Home and Health Department (Chief Scientist Organization, 1979). Commenting on differences in Scottish food consumption compared with the average for Great Britain, the working party emphasized the need for analysis of the diets of randomly selected small groups of the Scottish population in areas of contrasting rates of ischemic heart disease mortality and socioeconomic opportunity. They regarded dietary analysis methodology as of critical importance and proposed utilizing the more recent tables on food consumption that include new items such as vegetable fiber and polyunsaturated fatty acid as a means of producing more accurate dietary studies by computer. They recommended prospective recording of a week's food and drink intake supported by appropriate laboratory procedures, including such techniques as the analysis of adipose tissue samples to permit dietary fat saturation level assessment.

The review of nutritional assessment in health programs that emerged from the Proceedings of the Conference on Nutritional Assessment (1972), sponsored by the American Public Health Association in 1972, refers to pathological evidence of frank atherosclerosis in the arteries of young Americans in Korea and Vietnam as indicating the need for earlier identification of nutritional factors that may be disease precursors. In underlining the need for nutritional studies in cardiovascular disease, obesity, stroke, diabetes, and cancer, they draw attention to the possibility of certain foods and food additives being related to cancer of the gastrointestinal tract. Nutrition is also related to gout, hyperlipidemia, various anemias, intestinal enzyme deficiencies, alcoholism, arthritis, and accidents.

They delineate four major nutritional classifications to which nutrition may contribute: those with an excessive intake of calories or certain nutrients (usually carbohydrates); those with deficiencies of essential nutrients or calories; those with special nutritional problems, such as those occurring in diseases like ulcerative colitis, regional ileitis, alcoholism; and those with nonnutritional problems. They point to the need for guidelines to determine the extent of malnutrition (in itself an outcome) and its outcomes and for a broad system of dietary, clinical, and biochemical data collection.

At a basic level, information on an on-going epidemiological approach to cardiovascular disease involving nutrition is still available in the Tecumseh Study (Metzner *et al.*, 1977; Nichols *et al.*, 1976a,b), where stratified random samples of approximately 4,000 males and females between the ages of 19 and 25 years in a general population who had been clinically examined in 1960 had a dietary assessment in 1967. A card sort of 110 foods determined frequency, and a subsample in 2,000 participants completed 24-hour dietary recall. Adiposity was related to diet and food frequency to cholesterol. The study is prospective and may be expected to yield cumulative outcome data based on mortality. More frequent food intake appeared to be associated with less obesity.

CANCER METHODS

Morgan and his colleagues (Morgan *et al.*, 1978) evaluated three methods of estimating group and individual diet consumption in a case control study of diet in breast cancer. Their review of previous work in which nutritional methods were applied to epidemiological problems excluded the collection of nutrient data by methods requiring weighing and laboratory analysis as impractical for survey research. They restricted consideration to methods useful for field investigations aimed at identifying the dietary characteristics of large groups.

As in general methods of cardiovascular disease, the methods included the food frequency interview and inquiries about usual intake in terms of frequency of consumption of various food items, a method considered by Graham and his colleagues (Graham *et al.,* 1967) in a study of diet and gastric cancer as the most feasible approach giving a mean reliability of 81 percent.

Use of the quantitative research dietary history developed by Burke to record the subject's usual pattern of eating, as used in the Framingham Study where the interview was not structured, was considered to have failed to elicit all the required information. The Israel Ischaemic Heart Disease Study (Abramson *et al.,* 1963) also was not supportive of this method.

The diet record of foods and beverages consumed by the respondents was directly related to current intake, but was restricted to use by literate people.

Three days was regarded as the minimum time for a fair picture of food intake of the individual. The diet recall interview for the 24-hour period was believed to give fairly reliable data on current food consumption of a group. In their evaluation, the authors compare the efficacy of 24-hour recall, detailed quantitative diet history directed towards the most recent 2-month period after diagnosis and the 2-month period 6 months before diagnosis, and a 4-day diet diary. They found in this case control study of diet and breast cancer a high degree of correlation between the estimates of food consumption for the controls using each of the three methods. The highest estimate was obtained from diet history, with a slightly higher estimate in the period 6 months before diagnosis than in the current period. The lowest estimate was in 24-hour recall. They concluded that all three methods were applicable to case control studies, but diet history was preferred when current food intake may be influenced by a disease—frequently the case in cancer.

A closer examination of the methodology of nutritional assessment in relation to cancer is provided by a review of diet and breast cancer by Jean Hankin and her colleague (Hankin and Rawlings, 1978). Their review emphasizes the need for methodology to encompass the usual demographic factors and relate diet to outcome in high and low geographic areas of prevalence. The need to assess the possiblity of tumor initiation or inhibition in relation to diet, nutritional status, and hormonal pattern for and during teenage years is proposed, as well as the need to include genetic and environmental factors in studies of families who share genes as well as common environmental factors, including food intake. The excess of estrogen in obese women is considered a factor, although there has been no consistency between obesity measures and breast cancer. Weight and height individually were risk factors in prospective breast cancer study in women aged 55 to 74 years, but the association was weaker using the Quetelet's index (weight per height) (Marr, 1973). Height only was found constant for all risk attributable to body size.

Geographical variations are dealt with by correlation of breast cancer incidence with dietary and other environmental variables on a per capita basis, principally in relation to fat intake. In one study sugar was positively correlated and starch negatively correlated in per capita nutrient intakes in 10 countries with cancer mortality in single and married women. The per capita food and nutrient intakes were reported by the Food and Agricultural Organization (FAO) of the United Nations and were based on estimates of domestic food production, imports and exports, military supplies, and changes in stocks and reserves. Standard food composition values were then applied. These food estimates only reflect the amounts available per person and not the quantities consumed. The distribution of food by sex and age within the country are not described.

Studies of cancer rates in ethnic groups are helpful in formulating hypotheses. Breast cancer in first- and second-generation Japanese women living in San Francisco compared with Japan incriminate increased intakes of fat and its nutritional correlates. Stocks (1970) examined the regional variation of breast cancer death rates in England and Wales and the higher rates in the South compared with the North of Wales using per capita food intakes from annual national food surveys and cancer mortality. He found positive associations between milk, butter, and cheese and negative associations between other fats such as margarine. Nutrient intakes were not reported. Food frequency was collected from 100,000 Seventh Day Adventists in California and followed for 4 years by Philips (1975): 77 breast cancer cases were each matched by age, sex, and race with three controls from the study population. Comparison of the case-control dietary data showed that the frequencies of eating 5 food items were associated with breast cancer: fried potatoes, hard fat (butter, margarine, or shortening) for frying, all fried foods, dairy products except milk, and white bread. Relative risks ranged from 2.6 to 1.6. It was considered difficult, however, to draw inferences from qualitative food frequencies.

Quantitative data were used in a case control study in Canada where Miller (1977) collected data on usual intakes of participants. Mean nutrient intakes in 309 matched pairs showed difference in calories and total and saturated fats significantly higher among cases than controls.

In mice it has been suggested that tumorigenesis inhibited through a 30 percent reduction in calories is due to lack of energy (Tannenbaum, 1942), or possibly through pituitary insufficiency leading to a decrease of estrogen production and lower sensitivity leading to a decrease of estrogen production and lower sensitivity of breast cancer to estrogenic stimuli (Huseby *et al.*, 1945). In animal experiments, a one-third reduction in calories was necessary for tumor inhibition, but it is possible that inadequate calories and undernutrition in many developing countries of Asia and Africa might explain their low incidence of breast cancer.

Hill and his colleagues found persons on high-fat diets had higher proportions of anaerobic bacteria in the intestinal microflora and secreted more biliary steroids than those in low-fat intakes (Hill *et al.*, 1971). These bacteria are able to synthesize estrogens such as estradiol and estrone, potentially carcinogenic to the breast.

In animal studies the inhibitory effects of diets low in protein or selected amino acids have been considered to be related to changes in the immunological system (Alcantara and Speckman, 1976). It has been hypothesized that cellular immunity is a major defense against cancer, whereas humeral (antibody) immunity enhances tumorigenesis by depressing cellular immune responses. It is suggested that a low-protein intake might suppress antibody production, but have no effect on cellular immunity. There has been little evidence that different amounts of vitamins and minerals influence the incidence of mammary tumors. Morris (1947), on the other hand, observed that a deficiency of riboflavin decreased the number and growth of tumors in mice, whereas a supplement increased incidence. This has been confirmed in other studies, but the mechanism is unknown.

MacMahon and his colleagues have reviewed hypotheses relating breast cancer to viruses, genetics, exogenous hormones, and radiation. Diet or nutritional status might function as a modifier of mammary tumorigenesis.

Sections of the review (Hankin and Rawlings, 1978) consider antigens, estrogens, and prolactin. It is concluded that human breast cancer is multifactorial and that it seems highly probable that dietary factors are related to the disease in several ways. Metabolism of nutrients, synthesis and activity of several hormones, and the role of fatty tissue may be common areas of interaction that might favor mammary carcinogenesis. Dietary studies in animals should not be extrapolated to humans.

The National Cancer Institute, National Institutes of Health, Diet, Nutrition and Cancer Program report (1977) identified diet as an etiologic factor distinct from dietary contaminants and from genetic and environmental factors as playing a prominent role in the causation of certain major forms of cancer on the basis of the correlation between incidence and dietary habits in numerous studies of migrant populations, high- and low-cancer incidence populations, and special population groups and by studies of trends in cancer incidence and diet habits in the United States, Japan, and other countries. The report concludes that the most likely clue to the etiology of colon and breast cancer is diet-dependent, because these conditions do not appear to be affected appreciably by environmental polluters, food contaminants, smoking, or occupational exposure. It is also considered that the epidemiological evidence is reinforced because many of the relationships have been found to apply to cardiovascular disease (Stamler *et al.*, 1972; Dayton and Pearce, 1969).

This hypothesis is supported by experimental evidence of dietary factors in which calorie restriction in animals generally inhibits dietary fat and promotes tumorigenesis in the pregenerative stage of hormone-dependent tumors (Carroll, 1975). Modan and his colleagues in Israel report a higher consumption of starches among gastric cancer patients and a lower fiber consumption among colon cancer patients (Modan *et al.*, 1975). World population studies are used by Lowenfels and Anderson (1977) to positively correlate dietary factors specifically with colon and gastric cancers. They describe total calorie intake, nutritional excess or deficit, exposure to carcinogens, and consumption of alcohol as contributory factors. Comparison of spouses of Japanese women with breast cancer was used to isolate environmental from dietary factors prospectively. The spouses of breast cancer cases consumed more beef or meat, butter/margarine/cheese, corn, and wieners than other men (Gutsch and Holler, 1975).

DIABETES METHODS

The role of diet in diabetes is uncertain in a situation in which treatment does not appear to prolong life expectancy.

The epidemology of diabetes in Europe is reviewed by Gutsch and Holler (1975), whose most important contribution has been extension of standarization recommendations to facilitate international comparisons, such as the collaborative studies of the relationship of glucose intolerance to cardiovascular mortality involving several countries reported by the Stamlers at the VIII World Congress of Cardiology at Tokyo, Japan, in September 1978.

Studies in North America would seem to indicate that the main role of diet in therapy was calorie restriction to reduce obesity in itself proposed together with genetic factors as the major risk factors, especially in the elderly (West, 1973). The reviewer reports studies whose methodologies compare nutrition and dietary patterns in Japan, Israel, and Africa and support a relationship with diet in his own studies in 11 countries and in a review of published data in New World aboriginals: Indians, Eskimos, Polynesians, and Micronesians. A major conclusion from a review of all available laboratory and epidemiological evidence identifies total calorie intake independent of source as the most important dietary factor in increasing the risk of diabetes.

OBESITY

The risk of ischemic heart disease associated with obesity is small compared with other factors (Prevention of coronary heart disease, 1976). When factors associated with obesity, like blood pressure, glucose intolerance or diabetes mellitus, physical activity, or raised plasma levels of triglycerides, cholesterol, and uric acid are held constant, the predictive value of obesity for ischemic heart disease is much reduced, suggesting that when obesity does increase morbidity or mortality it does so through these factors.

Use of obesity as an index of dietary intake, nutritional health or disease, and disability status requires provision in analyses for hypertension, hyperlipidaemia, and glucose intolerance, as well as morbidity from ischemic heart disease. Provision must be made for neuromuscular incoordination, accidents, respiratory and skin disorders, emotional problems, and also for a general increase in mortality.

Measurement of obesity requires definition of criteria and standardization of technique. If obesity-associated conditions can be provided for, obesity or overweight might have possibilities as an abbreviated and, dependent of criteria, a simple index of nutritional status. The importance of birth weight as an accurate index of short-term outcomes, with important heredity and nutritional implications in the epidemiological assessment of health status, cannot be overemphasized.

DISCUSSION

There seems to be agreement that weighing of food is too much to ask of participants in epidemiological surveys, but within certain limits (Madden *et al.*, 1976; Young *et al.*, 1952) reliance can be placed on a combination of estimated current record, 24-hour recall, and diet history adapted in frequency and extent to meet the design requirements of individual studies.

Quantitative assessments can be made, and the use of new food tables or tables prepared specifically by chemical analysis for individual studies can reduce error in deriving nutrient values. Qualitative data can be collected from food frequency studies, which may be restricted to specific foods in developing a scoring system.

Cross-sectional epidemiological studies can be used to relate different "cut points" in the distribution of food or nutrient intake to the prevalence of outcomes like nutritional status measured by physical examination of indices like height and weight or biochemistry taken at the time of collection of dietary data. Relative risks can be calculated from these data, but a method much to be preferred would be prospective, in which outcomes in different percentiles of baseline dietary intake can be measured over time against incidence outcomes like weight gain or loss in nutrition, incidence of angina, or ECG abnormality in morbidity or cardiac infarction, stroke, or cancer in mortality. Only in prospective studies can outcomes against baseline dietary distributions be used to calculate relative and attributable risks for the individual and attributable risk for the community with the requisite degree of accuracy.

When mortality incidence is required for chronic disease outcomes, the methodology requires Framingham (Kannel and Gordon, 1970) or Tecumseh-like (Metzner *et al.*, 1977; Nichols *et al.*, 1976) studies on a sufficiently large scale to produce enough deaths or major disabilities within a reasonable time interval. Sample size is increased in proportion to the need to adjust the statistical cells to provide for demographic factors like age and sex and confounding factors like smoking.

Medical record linkage may offer a possible solution to the resource difficulties of conventional population studies. The application of validated, *abbreviated* dietary recall (Hankin *et al.*, 1978) to random probability samples such as those developed for statewide telephone inquiry could provide baseline dietary data in a sample of 2,500, which could characterize a population of 10,000,000. Deficiencies could be reviewed by deployment of the resource represented by the First Health and Nutrition Examination Survey (1972). Linkage to death certifications, cancer registration, and morbidity such as hospital admission data available from CPHA (Wylie and Slee, 1979) could provide appropriate outcomes. The larger the sample, the shorter the time to acquire an adequate number of outcomes to calculate risk.

What seems to be needed in nutrition is a more comprehensive and integrated health intelligence service. An appropriate existing organization such as CDC might be encouraged to assume responsibility for a more active role in collection and surveillance of national statistics of health outcome in terms of mortality and morbidity having nutritional implications.

Access to existing computer tapes can provide mortality and morbidity for relevant ICD chronic disease classifications. These could be analyzed for the usual demographic variables by geographic area down to HSA's, thus providing a means of identifying high- and low-risk groups for more detailed study by telephone or other methods outlined above.

Equally, surveillance of various indices of infant mortality, together with birth certification data, including birth weight when studied in the same comprehensive way, could shorten the long observation periods needed to collect mortality and morbidity prospectively in adult populations. Fetal nutritional experience would seem to offer the only prospect of studying chronic disease within a realistic time cycle for most investigators. Although the permeability of the placental barrier has been adequately demonstrated over many years, the potential of fetal susceptibility and use of cordblood for surveillance has not yet been purposefully used.

The best deployment for federal dietary research resources (First Health and Nutrition Examination Survey, 1974; Owen, 1978) would seem to be in prospective studies of high- and low-risk populations identified by the surveillance procedure using appropriate combinations of the methodologies described in this paper. The relatively ineffectual nature of past contributions in large part stems from failure to attempt more than cross-sectional estimates of population samples under study. There is urgent need to review these practices and use these resources prospectively in high- and low-risk samples. Increased precision in correlating diet and nutrition to health status can best be obtained by observation of the same individual over time. A small national resource could economically and effectively acquire such extra detailed data as might be needed to complement data already available from existing sources. Creation of an integrated nutritional health intelligence service might be the best method of relating diet and nutrition to outcome in chronic disease. The overriding need would seem to be integration of responsibility.

REFERENCES

Abramson, J. H., C. Some, and C. Kosovsky. 1963. Food frequency interview as an epidemiological tool. Am. J. Public Health 53:1093–1101.

Alcantara, E. N., and E. W. Speckman. 1976. Diet, nutrition and cancer. Am. J. Clin. Nutr. 29:1035.

Becker, B. G., B. P. Indik, and A. M. Beeuwkes. 1960. Diet intake methodologies. Technical report. University of Michigan, Ann Arbor.

Burk, C. M., and E. M. Pao. 1976. Methodology for large-scale surveys of household and individual diets. Home Economics Research Report No. 40. Agricultural Research Service, Untied States Department of Agriculture, Washington, D.C.

Burke, B. S. 1947. The dietary history as a tool in research. J. Am. Diet. Assoc. 23:1041.

Carrol, K. K. 1975. Experimental evidence of dietary factors and hormone-dependent cancer. Cancer Res. 35:3502–3506.

Chief Scientist Organization. 1979. Report into coronary heart disease in Scotland. A report to the Chief Scientist by the Working Group on Ischaemic Heart Disease, Scottish Home and Health Department, Trinity Park House, Edinburgh, Scotland. pp. 8–9.

Dayton, S., and M. L. Pearce. 1969. Prevention of coronary heart disease and other complications of atherosclerosis by modified diet. Am. J. Med. 46:751.

Diet, nutrition and cancer program. 1977. National Cancer Institute, National Institutes of Health Status Report.

First Health and Nutrition Examination Survey, United States, 1971–1972. 1974. Dietary intake and biochemical findings. U.S. Department of Health, Education, and Welfare, Public Health Service, Health Resources Administration, National Center for Health Statistics, Rockville, Md.

Graham, S., A. M. Lilienfeld, and J. E. Tidings. 1967. Dietary and purgation factors in the epidemiology of gastric cancer. Cancer 20:2224–2234.

Gutsch H., and H. D. Holler. 1975. Diabetes epidemiology in Europe. Georg Thieme Publishers, Stuttgart.

Hankin, J. H., and M. S. Rawlings. 1978. Diet and breast cancer: A review. Am. J. Clin. Nutr. 31:2005–2016.

Hankin, J. H., V. Rawlings, and A. Nomura. 1978. Methods in nutrition. Am. J. Clin. Nutr. 31:355–359.

Hill, M. J., P. Goddard, and R. E. O. Williams. 1971. Gut bacteria and aetiology of cancer of the breast. Lancet 2:472.

Huseby, R. A., Z. B. Ball, and M. B. Visscher. 1945. Further observation on the influence of simple calorie restriction on mammary cancer incidence and related phenomena in C3H mice. Cancer Res. 5:40.

Kannel, W. B., and T. Gordon. 1970. The Framingham Study, an epidemiological investigation of cardiovascular disease. Section 24 (circulated).

Keen H., and G. A. Rose. 1958. Diet and arterial disease in a population sample. Br. Med. J. 1:1508.

Lowenfels, A. B., and M. E. Anderson. 1977. Diet and cancer. Cancer 39:1809–1814.

Madden, J. P., S. J. Goodman, and H. A. Guthrie. 1976. Validity of the 24-hour recall. Research 68:143–147.

Marr, J. W. 1973. Dietary survey methods: Individual and group aspects. Proc. R. Soc. Med. 66:639–641.

Metzner, H. L., D. E. Lamphiear, N. C. Wheeler, and F. A. Larkin. 1977. The relationship between frequency of eating and adiposity in adult men and women in the Tecumseh Community Health Study. Am. J. Clin. Nutr. 30:712–715.

Miller, A. B. 1977. Role of nutrition in the etiology of breast cancer. Cancer 39:2704.

Modan, B., V. Barell, F. Lubin, and M. Modan. 1975. Dietary factors and cancer in Israel. Cancer Res. 35:3503–3506.

Morgan, R. W., M. Jain, A. B. Miller, N. W. Choi, L. Mathews, L. Munen, J. D. Burch, J. Feather, G. R. Howe, and A. Kelly. 1978. A comparison of dietary methods in epidemiologic studies. Am. J. Epidmiol.6(107):488–498.

Morris, H. P. 1947. Effects on the genesis and growth of tumors associated with vitamin intake. Ann. N.Y. Acad. Sci. 49:119.

Nichols, A. B., C. Ravenscoft, D. E. Lamphiear, and L. D. Ostrander. 1976a. Independence of serum lipid levels and dietary habits: The Tecumseh Study. JAMA 17(236):1948–1953.

Nichols, A. B., C. Ravenscoft, D. F. Lamphiear, and L. D. Ostrander. 1976b. Daily nutritional intake and serum lipid levels: The Tecumseh Study. Am. J. Clin. Nutr. 29:1384–1392.

Owen, A. Y., 1978. Community nutrition in preventive health care services: A critical review of the literature. U.S. Department of Health, Education, and Welfare, U.S. Government Printing Office, Washington, D.C.

Philips, R. L. 1975. Role of life-style and diet habits in risk of cancer among Seventh-Day Adventists. Cancer Res. 35:3513.

Prevention of coronary heart disease. 1976. Report of a joint working party of the Royal College of Physicians of London and the British Cardiac Society. J. R. Coll. Phys. 3(10).

Proc. of Conference on Nutritional Assessment. 1972. Nutritional assessment in health programs. Am. J. Public Health 63:64.

Rose, G. A., and H. Blackburn. 1968. Cardiovascular survey methods. WHO Monograph Series No. 56. WHO, Geneva.

Stocks, P. 1970. Breast cancer anomalies. Br. J Cancer 24:633.

Stamler, J., D. M. Berleson, and H. A. Lindberg. 1972. Pages 41–119 in R. W. Wissler and J. C. Geer, eds. The pathogenesis of arteriosclerosis. Williams and Willins, Baltimore.

Tannenbaum, A. 1942. The genesis and growth of tumors. II. Effects of calorie restriction per se. Cancer Res. 2:460.

West, K. M. 1973. Prevention and therapy of diabetes mellitus. Nutr. Rev. 7:193–197.

Wylie, C. M., and V. N. Slee. 1979. Community health surveillance through hospital discharges. Univ. Mich. Med. Center J. 2(44):60–64.

Young, C. M., G. C. Hagan, R. E. Tucker, and W. D. Foster. 1952. A comparison of dietary study methods. II. Dietary history vs. seven-day record vs. 24-hour recall. J. Am. Diet. Assoc. 28:218–221.

Anthropometry and Nutritional Status

FRANCIS E. JOHNSTON

"Nutritional status" is a widely used term, usually employed in some fashion by almost anyone discussing the relationship between diet and health. Yet, despite its ubiquitous nature, definitions of nutritional status are difficult to find. Some use it epidemiologically to estimate the prevalence of malnutrition in a population, while others use it clinically to refer to the nutritional well-being of an individual. On the one hand, there are those who focus upon dietary intake in evaluating nutritional status, while on the other, there are those who rely upon indicators of disease as evidence for disturbances in status.

I will use nutritional status to refer to the extent to which the dietary intake has been sufficient to satisfy the nutrient needs. I will also use the term interchangeably to indicate the evaluation of an individual as well as the assessment of an entire group. While I realize that this is a global definition, lacking perhaps in specificity, the choice of the definition is dictated by the topic being discussed, as well as by the orientation of this workshop.

Clearly, such a broad definition demands a comprehensive set of techniques of assessment, in fact, a battery of techniques that will transcend any single discipline. While a single set of methods, e.g., biochemical, can yield a picture of nutritional status, and quite possibly one that is sufficient for the immediate purpose, the complete picture requires a broader approach.

Anthropometry, traditionally located within the history of physical anthropology, provides one set of methods and techniques, though only one of many (*see,* e.g., Jelliffe, 1966; Christakis, 1973; Guthrie, 1975). If I appear to be overselling anthropometry, it is because my task for this workshop is to indicate its usefulness. I hope also to indicate the limitations on anthropometry as a technique, one of several that are utilized in research and in assessment.

As a physical anthropologist, I do feel that anthropometry has not yet received its "just due" as a technique for assessing nutritional status. Part of that has come about because of the speckled history of anthropometry even within anthropology. But part of the blame must also rest upon our fascination, in Western culture, for methods developed in the experimental laboratory and in hospitals, and for the assumption that the methods developed in those settings could be exported into the surrounding community, or, worse yet, the remote communities of the nation and the world.

Thus, anthropometry is one of the basic techniques for the comprehensive assessment of nutritional status. The information provided by the careful measurement of the body cannot be obtained reliably by any other method. Likewise, the information provided by anthropometric data is valid within the constraints of the method, and, regardless of our wishes, we cannot push body measurements beyond those constraints, no matter how intently we wish or how elaborately we analyze our measurements.

ANTHROPOMETRY AS AN INDICATOR OF NUTRITIONAL STATUS

The term nutritional anthropometry began first to appear after World War II, but seems to have had its first significant impact with the publication of *Body Measurements and Human Nutrition,* edited by Josef Brozek (1956), the proceedings of a conference sponsored by the National Research Council. In his introduction to that volume, Brozek began to establish the link that forms the foundation for my discussion, namely, that body morphology—size, shape, and composition—reflects the dietary history of an individual and is an indicator of the adequacy of that history, or, in other words, of nutritional status. Accepting that, one central task of the conference was to determine a minimum number of measurements that could provide an estimate of nutritional status, selected from the countless number religiously measured by 250 years of anthropologists. This list has been updated in subsequent years as ensuing research has validated some, invalidated others, and developed still newer ones. A number of additional conferences, seminars, and workshops have concerned themselves with this task, and their deliberations have been duly reported in various publications (World Health Organization, 1968; McKigney and Munroe, 1976).

The Advantages of Anthropometry

The use of anthropometry in assessing nutritional status offers certain advantages. Some of these advantages are biological, i.e., they provide unique information, while others are practical.

First of all, anthropometry provides information on past nutritional history, information that is of value and that cannot be obtained with equal confidence using other techniques. In a more elegant way, we may say that one's nutritional history is embedded in his or her morphology and that this history is revealed through the analysis of measurements of that morphology. The analysis of body measurements can assist in the identification not only of severe states of malnutrition, but also of the mild-to-moderate malnutrition that we all suspect is so widespread, but that is more difficult to document than might be imagined.

Next, anthropometry is a relatively "easy" technique to employ, since it is noninvasive and applicable to situations where large sample sizes are desirable. Anthropometric equipment is generally portable and relatively inexpensive, requiring no portable generators, refrigerators, centrifuges, or autoclaves. While considerably more technician training is required than many scientists believe, a few months of careful training and some system of monitoring continued technical performance will suffice to provide a body of data with acceptably low errors of measurement.

The Limitations of Anthropometry

Anthropometric techniques do not provide a panacea, and anyone using it must be aware of its limitations. They reduce its comprehensiveness as a means of evaluating nutritional status and affect the accuracy of the data obtained.

Anthropometry provides only limited information on present nutritional status. While it is true that one's present status is a function of past nutritional intake, nonetheless, anthropometry is not able to detect short-term, nutrient-specific disturbances in nutritional status.

Second, while body morphology is indeed sensitive to nutritional disturbances, it is similarly altered by a variety of such disturbances; anthropometric indicators are not specific. Nutritional status may be altered adversely by any number of factors, primary as well as secondary. Careful measurement of the body will reveal that something has indeed gone adrift, and, if the limiting nutrient is already suspected, anthropometry can quantify the degree of nutritional insult, especially if it involves protein or energy. But body measurements will be much less likely to identify a deficiency or excess of a more specific nutrient, a vitamin or mineral. Furthermore, anthropometry may indicate simply that the morphology has been altered, but we may be uncertain whether the alteration is a direct result of malnutrition, or perhaps of some concomitant of malnutrition such as infectious disease, or in the case of overnutrition, of reduced energy expenditure.

Finally, anthropometry, in the classic sense, deals only with the surface of the body. Even though techniques such as radiogrammetry and ultrasonics may sometimes be subsumed under the general term "anthropometry," such is seldom the case in nutritional surveys. While the noninvasive nature of anthropometry is a decided asset, it also means that the measurements made are indirect. Their validity rests upon research that relates morphological alterations to underlying physiological processes to an extent that yields statistically reliable results.

Advantages and Limitations: One and the Same

A comparison of the foregoing reveals that, in fact, the advantages of anthropometry are its limitations. The reasons for adopting anthropometry in assessing nutritional status provide limitations upon its usefulness. The solution seems to be to judge the results of this trade-off, exploiting anthropometric data fully when the trade-off is not detrimental. The setting in which the assessment is to be made, the extent of data to be collected, and the use to which the assessments are to be put, all determine the methods eventually chosen.

Anthropometry seems especially appropriate when there is a suspected chronic imbalance of protein and energy. Such imbalances are known to distort the normal proportions of body tissues and to alter the patterns of physical growth, often quite drastically. These alterations become fixed, as it were, and may be identified during the adult years, long after growth has ceased. Thus, nutritional status changes may be evaluated from one generation to the next, analyzing the phenomenon known as the secular trend (Malina, 1979).

The Rationale for Nutritional Anthropometry

The initial step in establishing a rationale for nutritional anthropometry has been given above: Variations in the ratio between nutrient intake and nutrient requirement are recorded in the morphology of the body, perhaps permanently. The greater the disparity, the greater the morphological alterations, reaching the extremes of obesity and marasmus.

Taking this position to the extreme would require us to accept that all variation in body morphology results from variation in the ratio of intake to need. While there may be some extremists who hold this view, it seems to be an easy one to disprove. Nutritional factors are important determinants of our size, shape, and composition, but others may also be demonstrated: heredity, for example. Fortunately for our purposes, it seems that hereditary factors determining body morphology may be rather easily overridden by chronic nutritional disturbances. Mueller (1975), for example, has demonstrated that heritability estimates, derived from parent–offspring correlations, decrease as the prevalence of undernutrition increases. At the same time, different parameters show differential susceptibility. Body shape, or proportion, seems particularly resistant to nutritional variation (Tanner, 1978), and we would expect to find it altered only under the most stringent alterations of the diet.

Another aspect of the rationale for anthropometry is that body measurement may indicate the presence of malnutrition, even though a particular dimension may not itself be affected by the malnutrition that is detected. In humans, malnutrition, either over or under, seldom occurs in splendid isolation, but rather exists as part of an ecological complex. Undernutrition is almost always found where there is poverty, infectious disease, and crowding (Cravioto, 1970). Deficient fat and muscle stores, small body size, and delayed growth will characterize the inhabitants of such ecosystems, and, while we may not be able to specify how much of a given morphological deviation is directly produced by malnutrition, the greater the deviations from the normal, the greater the prevalence and the severity of the malnutrition. In other words, anthropometry may be, in many instances, not an effect, but an indicator.

Thus, the rationale for anthropometry as one component of the assessment of nutritional status is rooted in these two postulates. First, alterations in the intake/need ratio will be recorded in morphology. Second, the interrelationships of factors in a nutritional ecosystem will make anthropometry valuable as an indicator at the community level.

The selection of dimensions and the analysis of data is, in nutritional anthropometry, done within the context of two different schemes that, while not mutually exclusive, are to some extent independent. These schemes are (1) the measurement of growth and (2) the measurement of body composition.

The Measurement of Growth

Nutrient requirements, relative to body weight, are highest during the growing years, due to the additional nutrients needed to support body growth. Although reliable estimates of the requirements for growth are few, available evidence suggests that, during infancy, the energy necessary for growth may be as much as one-third that necessary for maintenance (Payne and Waterlow, 1977).

There is no doubt that the cost of undernutrition is highest for infants and preschool children exceeding, so it would seem, the cost among adults of overnutrition. Consequently, the effects of malnutrition upon the growth process are marked and often dramatic, and the growth patterns of the children of a population provide perhaps the best evidence of the general level of health of that population (Eveleth and Tanner, 1976). Van Duzen *et al.* (1976) have presented compelling evidence for this in their analysis of the increased growth among Navajo preschoolers in conjunction with the initiation of a feeding program. Not only did severe protein–energy malnutrition drop dramatically in its incidence, so did the heights and weights of the children increase.

Observations of individual children in response to dietary therapy or nutritional supplementation also provide evidence of the close relationship between growth and nutritional intake. Ashworth (1969) has described the sharp increases in the rates of growth of children from Jamaica who were recovering from PEM, while Lampl *et al.* (1978) documented a general, and statistically significant, increase in growth among chronically undernourished Papua New Guinean children whose diets were supplemented with a skimmed milk powder, compared to their age peers whose diets were not supplemented.

Because of the sensitivity of growth to nutritional deficiencies and excesses, the analysis of the growth records of children is widely used in evaluating nutritional status. There is, by now, ample evidence of the growth-retarding effects of undernutrition, especially of protein and energy, manifested in small body size, reduced fat stores, and deficient stores of muscle, as well as delays in the rate of biological maturation. Overnutrition is associated with increased deposition of adipose fat, accelerated rates of maturation, and possibly increased stature and lean body mass.

Some researchers have suggested that decreased growth in stature and muscle mass is indicative of a deficiency of protein, while decreased fat stores reflect energy insufficiency. However, this is not well supported by the available evidence and, given the fact that energy seems to be the nutrient that, on a worldwide basis, is limiting (Behar, 1977), it seems premature to utilize nutritional anthropometry in such a specific way at present.

Measurements of growth are especially well-suited for detecting children who have been subject to chronic mild-to-moderate malnutrition. Anthropometry can reveal this deficit, especially among children older than 12 months of age, when the cumulative effects of nutritional deficits become significantly registered in their morphology.

The Measurement of Body Composition

Three decades of intensive research have by now revealed that it is possible to separate analytically the mass of the human body into its component parts (see, e.g., Keys and Grande, 1973). The conceptual model used for analysis will vary from researcher to researcher, but, at a bare minimum, we may conceive of body mass as consisting of a fat component and a component called the lean body mass. Quantitatively body weight may be thought of as the sum of body fat plus the lean body mass (LBM), so that, by knowing weight, we need only determine one of the components in order to be able to solve for the other.

Various techniques are available for estimating body composition in the laboratory. The most widely used of these techniques involve the determination of one of the three variables: (1) the body density, (2) the volume of intracellular water, or (3) the mass of potassium, determined from counting the radioactive isotope, K^{40}. From any one of these three variables, it is possible to compute a value for LBM or for fat as a percentage of weight.

Since the mid-1920's, physical anthropologists have sought to measure more than linear dimensions and have developed instruments and techniques for estimating underlying masses of fat, muscle, and bone. These anthropometrically determined values have been correlated with values estimated from laboratory procedures in attempts to validate anthropometry and to provide equations allowing the quantification of body composition (Brozek and Henschel, 1963; Malina, 1969).

Variations in the amounts and proportions of body fat and lean body mass are indicators of nutritional status. The fat depot is especially sensitive to deviations from optimal energy intake, while chronic undernutrition will be recorded in muscle wasting.

NUTRITIONAL ANTHROPOMETRY—A MINIMUM LIST

To suggest a minimum list of measurements to be used in assessing nutritional status is dangerous and possibly foolhardy. Different investigators will favor different measurements: Some will insist upon a lengthy list, while others will utilize but one or two. Despite this, it seems that, over the years, a certain consensus has emerged, at least insofar as a minimum set of dimensions is concerned. In this section, I wish to present my interpretation of that list. But I wish also to present a second list, consisting of a few additional measurements that will be of use in certain situations. The first list is, in my opinion, the bare minimum without which an adequate assessment of nutritional status based upon anthropometry cannot be done. The second list includes measurements that will be of value if other kinds of analysis are to be done, especially relating possible causative factors in the environment to body morphology.

The minimum list consists of the following dimensions:

1. body length (from 2 years on, standing height is to be measured);
2. head circumference;
3. body weight;
4. mid upper arm circumference;
5. triceps skinfold; and
6. subscapular skinfold.

The additions, referred to above as the second list, are as follows:

1. biacromial diameter (bony shoulder girdle);
2. bicristal diameter (bony pelvic girdle);
3. sitting height; and
4. suprailiac skinfold.

The procedures outlined in the Staff Training Manual of Cycle III of the U.S. Health Examination Survey (HES), represent the most comprehensive collection of health data, including anthropometry, perhaps ever collected in the world, and the various mensurational procedures were developed carefully and thoughtfully. However, other such sets of procedures are available, and, for those few measurements of the above lists not measured directly by the HES (stature and supine length), one should consult the handbook of the International Biological Program (IBP) (Weiner and Lourie, 1969).

It goes without saying that those taking the measurements must be well-trained, and even simple measurements such as height and weight cannot be approached naively. A big part of the problem of the validity of height and weight as measures of nutritional status has been the often-cavalier way they have been approached by clinicians, nurses, and public health workers. Anthropometry can give useful results, but only if the technicians involved are well-trained, utilize standard techniques, and undergo periodic training sessions to eliminate idiosyncratic factors, to reduce both systematic and random error, and to quantify the error of measurement.

In addition to the above measurements, three derivations from the raw data are recommended. First is an evaluation of weight-for-height. Or, alternatively, one may calculate the index: weight-(height)^2, known as Quetelet's index. Second is the calculation of the relative sitting height, sitting height/stature, a measure of the ratio of trunk (plus head) to leg length. Finally, the muscle mass of the body may be estimated by deriving the estimated circumference of the muscle of the upper arm, upper arm muscle circumference. Since both the upper arm circumference and the triceps skinfold are to be taken at the same level, the middle of the upper arm, and since the triceps skinfold is an estimate of the double layer of fat at that site (plus skin), if we asume that the arm and the underlying muscle are circular, the UAMC may be estimated as follows:

$$\text{UAMC} = (\text{Upper Arm Circumference}) - (\text{Triceps}).$$

While this may seem to involve a number of assumptions, as it does, it will be seen below that this measurement does have enough validity to warrant its use.

Reference Standards

One of the problems of nutritional anthropometry is that it requires standards against which to evaluate the data collected. After several years of discussion and debate, the majority of investigators now agree that it is impossible to specify true "norms" as standards. Instead it is now customary to use "reference standards" or "reference data" that provide a useful yardstick against which measurements may be compared.

At least two schools of thought exist regarding the selection of reference standards. First, there are those persons who advocate the use of local standards, derived from ethnically similar groups, to minimize genetic factors. Second, there are those who advocate the use of a single standard, drawn from some well-defined and accurately sampled population. Proponents of the single standard feel that the problem of genetic differences is minimized because of the advantages associated with one "universal" yardstick. My own sympathies are with the latter position, since the development of a large number of local standards, whatever local means, could very well lead to chaos.

It is generally agreed that the single best set of reference standards are those of the HES. For children, these standards have been highly refined, using sophisticated statistical procedures, and are currently published and distributed by Ross Laboratories. Since they are based upon national probability samples, and since they are as up-to-date as is possible, they are suitable not only for the United States, but also for reference use elsewhere. Unfortunately, only height and weight have been subjected to statistical smoothing, but the descriptive statistics are generally available for other measurements in the publications of the National Center for Health Statistics (NCHS).

Data on adults are not as satisfactory. Cycle I of the HES examined 18- to 74-year-olds, and the measurements were analyzed and published in the NCHS series. However, the Durvey was conducted in the early 1960's, and any secular trend could create problems. The successor to the HES, HANES, has examined all age-groups, and the results are beginning to appear. As these results are published, we will have adequate data on the entire age range to be examined.

THE VALIDITY OF NUTRITIONAL ANTHROPOMETRY

The utility of anthropometry in assessing nutritional status must ultimately rest upon its ability to predict individuals who are nutritionally at-risk, or to determine the existence of some degree of malnutrition in a specific group. This may be done in a number of ways, and, in fact, there is now a large literature on anthropometry as an indicator of nutritional status. A review of that literature is well beyond the scope of this paper, but it is worthwhile to point to some examples of research that have attempted to validate nutritional anthropometry.

We may begin with the consideration of the relationship between physical growth and malnutrition, and focus, for convenience, upon my own research. For about 5 years we have been analyzing the data collected by Joaquin Cravioto as part of his study of "The Land of the White Dust," in southern Mexico. We have collected additional data ourselves, and several publications have either appeared or are in press, resulting from our studies. In one such study, Scholl (1975) identified, from the cohort under study of over 280, a subgroup of 72 children who manifested failing growth between 6 months and 3 years of age. These children were hypothesized to be suffering from chronic undernutrition. Support for this came from our finding that, of the 19 children of the cohort subsequently hospitalized for severe protein–energy malnutrition, 14 came from this failing subgroup. Furthermore, of the seven children who died, between 12 and 60 months, of nutrition-related causes, 6 came from this failing subgroup. In other words, failing physical growth was effective at identifying children who were nutritionally at-risk.

Many other investigators have also established the link between reduced growth and malnutrition. In some instances, this link is used to identify individual children who may be singled out for therapy, while, in other cases, the measurement of growth may be used as an indicator of the existence of malnutrition in a community or a socioeconomic group.

Another aspect of the validity of anthropometry is its correlation with estimates of body composition determined physiologically. Since antrhopometry is localized and noninvasive, estimates of body composition are necessarily indirect. Despite this, there does seem to be agreement that body measurements, given the proper analysis, can estimate underlying tissue masses. Certainly the measurement of the triceps skinfold is often used as the best indicator of obesity, and certainly is much better than an index of weight-for-height.

TABLE 1 Partial Correlations (Age-Constant) of Anthropometry and Body Composition (Densitometry) in 12–17-Year-Olds

	Males	Females
Sample size	119	24
Arm muscle circ./LBM	0.778	0.629
Triceps skinfold/fat	0.838	0.741
Subscapular skinfold/fat	0.832	0.766

Table 1 presents some yet-unpublished data from a recent study of ours, in which we correlated, among 12- to 17-year-olds, anthropometric dimensions with LBM and body fat, estimated by densitometry. The correlations indicate that, among this sample, anthropometry can provide good estimates of these two variables, and, using more than simple bivariate correlations, considerable higher proportions of the variance in fat or LBM could be accounted for by body measurement. Again, research is still needed to establish the best use of the measurements, but the results seem quite promising.

To me there is little doubt that anthropometry provides useful measures of nutritional status, and, in certain situations, may be the method of choice. As I noted earlier, anthropometry is not the nutritional utopia that we all desire, but, used judiciously and wisely, it becomes an integral component. It is at its best when used in surveys and when used epidemiologically. When applied to individuals whose nutritional imbalance has not been chronic, it is not as accurate. For example, recently Young and Hill (1978) assessed changes in anthropometric dimensions of 54 adult patients undergoing surgery. They found anthropometry to be insensitive as an indicator of protein depletion in individuals. However, a reading of their paper reveals flaws in their methodology, which may or may not have detracted from their findings. In any event, it seems that anthropometry is not as useful in such conditions as are other indicators.

Anthropometry may be used to indicate parents who are at-risk of having children who will develop malnutrition or who may be especially susceptible to nutritional deficiency. Our research in Mexico indicates that the body sizes of the parents are the best indicators of children who display chronic malnutrition. In another study, Lechtig *et al.* (1976), of the INCAP, have found maternal stature, head circumference, and housing quality to be significant biosocial indicators of women more likely to produce a low birth-weight infant. The link to nutrition seems to be established, in this group, through the reduction in the incidence of low birth weights of women from the lowest socioeconomic groups (Lechtig *et al.*, 1975).

SUMMARY

Anthropometry is a much-abused yet time-honored technique. However, nutritional anthropometry is a dynamic methodology, in which measurements are being developed and applied to specific situations. The results are promising and suggest that body morphology is a sensitive indicator of malnutrition. Anthropometry cannot be employed haphazardly, uncritically, or without an understanding of the underlying theory relating body size and shape to body composition and growth and their alteration with malnutrition.

REFERENCES

Ashworth, A. 1969. Growth rates in children recovering from protein–calorie malnutrition. Br. J. Nutr. 23:835–845.

Behar, M. 1977. Protein-calorie deficits in developing countries. Ann. N.Y. Acad. Sci. 300:176–187.

Brozek, J., ed. 1956. Body measurements and human nutrition. Wayne State University Press, Detroit.

Brozek, J., and A. Henschel, ed. 1963. Techniques for measuring body composition. National Academy of Sciences–National Research Council, Washington, D.C.

Christakis, G., ed. 1973. Nutritional assessment in health programs. American Public Health Association, Washington, D.C.

Cravioto, J. C. 1970. Complexity of factors involved in protein–calorie malnutrition. Bibl. Nutr. Dieta 14:7–22.

Eveleth, P. B., and J. M. Tanner. 1976. Worldwide variation in human growth. Cambridge University Press, New York.

Guthrie, H. A. 1975. Introductory nutrition. C. V. Mosby, St. Louis.

Jelliffe, D. B. 1966. The assessment of the nutritional status of the community. WHO, Geneva.

Keys, A. F., and F. Grande. 1973. Body weight, body composition, and calorie status. *In* R. S. Goodhart and M. E. Shils, eds. Modern nutrition in health and disease. Lea and Febiger, Philadelphia.

Lampl, M., F. E. Johnston, and L. A. Malcolm. 1978. The effects of protein supplementation on the growth and skeletal maturation of New Guinean schoolchildren. Ann. Human Biol. 5:219–228.

Lechtig, A., H. Delgado, R. E. Lasky, R. E. Klein, P. L. Engle, C. Yarbrough, and J-P. Habicht. 1975. Maternal nutrition and fetal growth in developing societies: Socioeconomic factors. Am. J. Dis. Child. 129:434–437.

Lechtig, A., H. Delgado, C. Yarbrough, J-P. Habicht, R. Martorell, and R. E. Klein. 1976. A simple assessment of the risk of low birth weight to select women for nutritional intervention. Am. J. Obstet. Gynecol. 125:25–34.

McKigney, J. I., and H. N. Munroe, ed. 1976. Nutrient requirements in adolescence. MIT Press, Cambridge, Mass.

Malina, R. M. 1969. Quantification of fat, muscle, and bone in man. Clin. Orthoped. 65:9–38.

Malina, R. M. 1979. Secular changes in size and maturity: Causes and effects. In A. F. Roche, ed. Monogr. Soc. Ref. Child Dev., in press.

Mueller, W. H. 1975. Parent–child and sibling correlations and heritability of body measurement in a rural Colombian population. Ph.D. Dissertation, University of Texas, Austin.

Payne, P. R., and J. C. Waterlow, 1977. Relative energy requirements for maintenance, growth, and physical activity. Lancet 2:210–211.

Scholl, T. O. 1975. Body size in developing nations: Is bigger better? PhD. Dissertation. Temple University, Philadelphia.

Tanner, J. M. 1978. Foetus into man: Physical growth from conception to maturity. Harvard University Press, Cambridge, Mass.

Van Duzen, J., J. P. Carter, and R. V. Zwagg. 1976. Oritein and calorie malnutrition among preschool Navajo children: A follow-up. Am. J. Clin. Nutr. 29:657–662.

Weiner, J. S., and J. A. Lurie. 1969. Human biology: A guide to field methods. IBP Handbook No. 9. F. A. Davis, Philadelphia.

World Health Organization. 1968. Nutritional status of populations: A manual on anthropometric appraisal of trends. WHO/Nutr/70.129. WHO, Geneva.

Young, G. A., and G. L. Hill. 1978. Assessment of protein–calorie malnutrition in surgical patients from plasma proteins and anthropometric measurements. Am. J. Clin. Nutr. 31:429–435.

Relation of Nutritional Anemias to Food Consumption Patterns

VICTOR HERBERT

SUMMARY

The American diet is marginal in absorbable iron content for infants and children under age 5, for children at the growth spurt of puberty, and for women in the child-bearing years. Folate deficiency is common among people not eating each day one fresh or fresh-frozen uncooked fruit or vegetable or fruit juice. Vitamin B_{12} deficiency is common on a dietary basis only among pure vegetarians.

Iron-deficiency anemia and folate (folic acid) deficiency anemia are more common in women than men both because of the monthly loss of these two nutrients in blood during the menstrual years and the taking up of these nutrients by the fetus at the expense of the mother during pregnancy. During the menstrual years, because of the monthly blood loss, women have approximately twice the daily iron need of men. For them, the American diet is marginal in iron, and approximately 40 to 50 percent of premenopausal women may have iron depletion and about 15 percent have iron-deficiency anemia. After age 50, only about 13 percent of women have iron depletion. Iron depletion is present in about 50 percent of infants and iron-deficiency anemia in about 25 percent. Iron depletion is present in about 10 percent of children at the growth spurt of puberty.

Both the Committee on Maternal Nutrition (1970) and the Committee on Dietary Allowances (1974) of the Food and Nutrition Board, National Research Council recommend that folic acid and iron supplements should be taken throughout pregnancy. The Committee on Dietary Allowances recommendation was that the recommended dietary allowance be doubled in pregnancy, to 800 μg daily. Data presented at the 1975 Folate Workshop of the National Academy of Sciences suggest that such an amount could not easily be achieved without supplementation. Oral contraceptives reduce monthly blood loss, thereby reducing the frequency of iron deficiency. The question of whether the existing iron fortification of American flour should be increased (AMA Council on Foods and Nutrition, 1972: Wintrobe, 1973) has been decided in the negative on grounds of inadequate information to make an adequate risk:benefit assessment. In this connection, it should be noted that American breads are now mainly fortified with ferrous sulfate, with a trend to ferrum reductum, and American spaghettis and pastas with the less absorbable ferrous pyrophosphate (Dudley Titus, personal communication). Canada requires that more than 90 percent of ferrum reductum fortification be the more absorbable less than 10 micron particle size, but the United States has no size requirements.

Several surveys have shown lower serum and red cell folate in women taking oral contraceptives, but a daily fresh uncooked vegetable, fruit, or fruit juice would probably prevent folate deficiency in this group as well as many other groups.

INTRODUCTION

Anemia is defined as a reduction below normal in the amount of red blood that occurs when the equilibrium between blood production and loss (through bleeding or destruction) is disturbed *(Dorland's Illustrated Medical Dictionary,* 1974). By World Health Organization criteria (1968; Baker and DeMaeyer, 1979), anemia is considered to exist when the nonpregnant adult female has a hemoglobin below 12 and the pregnant adult female a hemoglobin below 11 g/100 ml of venous blood (when at sea level; normal values are higher at higher altitudes). The observations of Scott *et al.* (1970) indicate that the hemoglobin concentration of healthy nonpregnant young women without iron deficiency will almost always be 12 g/100 ml or more, that at mid-pregnancy this value will practically always be at least 10 g/100 ml, but fairly often may be less than 11 g/100 ml, and late in pregnancy this figure will almost always be 10 g/100 ml or more, and most often 11 g/100 ml or more, in the absence of iron deficiency. The normal fall of hemoglobin during pregnancy is simply pregnancy hypervolemia (which increases both the plasma and red cell volume, with a greater increase in the former).

Nutritional anemia is defined as a condition in which the hemoglobin content of the blood is lower than normal as a result of deficiency of one or more essential nutrients. To delineate a given anemia as nutritional, two criteria must be met: lack of the nutrient must produce, and providing the nutrient must correct, the anemia. By these two criteria, there are only three unequivocal nutritional anemias: those due to lack of iron, folate, or vitamin B_{12} (Herbert, 1970). These three anemias reflect an important nutritional problem affecting large population groups, particularly the poverty-stricken and those under metabolic stress.

Iron deficiency and folate deficiency are more common in women because of two forms of metabolic stress peculiar to women: the monthly blood loss in premenopausal women and the drain on maternal nutrient stores imposed by pregnancy. The fetus will take from the mother whatever it needs in order to be born normal, even if this produces severe nutrient deficiency in the mother (Committee on Maternal Nutrition, 1970). Since anemia is a relatively late manifestation of nutritional deficiency, those patients diagnosed as having nutritional anemia are the "tip of the iceberg"—part of a larger group suffering from nutrient depletion of more moderate degree, which is not yet manifest by unequivocal anemia.

The metabolic stress of menstrual blood loss is increased by the use of some intrauterine contraceptive devices (Anonymous, 1974, 1975) and decreased by the use of oral contraceptives (Anonymous, 1973). In fact, advertising of "unique vitamin–mineral formulas for the special needs of patients taking oral contraceptives" are misleading because it has not been established that there is any such special need (Anonymous, 1973; Symposium, 1975).

IRON-DEFICIENCY ANEMIA

Fairbanks *et al.* (1971) tabulated the approximate frequency of iron depletion as 50 percent of infants, 50 percent of premenopausal women, and 100 percent of pregnant women. They tabulated the frequency of iron-deficiency anemia (the end product of prolonged iron depletion) as 25 percent of infants, 0–5 percent of children (higher frequency was in economically deprived children), 15 percent of premenopausal women, and 30 percent of pregnant women not receiving iron supplementation.

About one-third to one-half of apparently healthy young American women have laboratory evidence of iron depletion (Monsen *et al.*, 1967; Scott and Pritchard, 1967; Sturgeon and Shoden, 1971). Sturgeon and Shoden (1971) found less than 5 mg of iron/100 g liver tissue in 40 percent of women age 20 to 50, indicative of iron depletion. This was true of only 13 percent of women over age 50 (and less than 10 percent of all men). It should be noted that iron depletion (loss of body iron stores) precedes anemia. While a majority of women who are anemic have iron deficiency, this is not always the case, so self-administration of medicinal iron may be unwise, and blanket treatment of every anemic woman with iron, without ascertaining that she, in fact, has iron deficiency, can do positive harm (as, for example, in women with sickle-cell or other hemolytic anemias with increased iron stores, in whom the giving of iron may produce "iron overload" syndrome). Nevertheless, the incidence of anemia in various groups of pregnant American women has ranged from 10 to 60 percent, most of which could be prevented by prophylactic iron therapy (AMA Council on Foods and Nutrition, 1968).

Menstrual loss of iron is the main source of the iron losses in nonpregnant women in the fertile age-group (Rybo, 1970; Fairbanks *et al.,* 1971). The average menstrual blood loss is about 40 ml/cycle (Fairbanks *et al.,* 1971), representing a loss of about 20 mg of iron per cycle. About 10 percent of women have menorrhagia, with a blood loss exceeding 80 ml/cycle (Hallberg *et al.,* 1966), making them particularly susceptible to iron deficiency. The use of more than 12 pads during a menstrual period, of the damming up of blood behind tampons, often suggests excessive menstrual bleeding (More and Dubach, 1956: Fairbanks *et al.,* 1971).

An understanding of the situation of American women with respect to iron balance is more clearly made by reference to Tables 1 and 2, which present respectively the estimated dietary iron requirements of Americans (Table 1) and the iron requirements of pregnant American women (Table 2). The absorbability of iron from different food sources is highly variable, averaging out to about 10 percent of iron in the total diet being absorbed (Layrisse, 1975; Cook, 1978). Therefore, the amount of iron ingested must be 10-fold

TABLE 1 Estimated Dietary Iron Requirements

	Absorbed Iron Requirement, mg/day	Dietary Iron Requirement,[a] mg/day
Normal men and nonmenstruating women	0.5–1.0	5–10
Menstruating women	0.7–2.0	7–20
Pregnant women	2.0–4.8	20–48[b]
Adolescents	1.0–2.0	10–20
Children	0.4–1.0	4–10
Infants	0.5–1.5	1.5 mg/kg[c]

[a] Assuming 10 percent absorption.

[b] This amount of iron cannot be derived from diet and should be met by iron supplementation in the latter half of pregnancy.

[c] To a maximum of 15 mg.

SOURCE: After Council on Foods and Nutrition, 1968. Courtesy of the *Journal of the American Medical Association*.

TABLE 2 Iron Requirements for Pregnancy

	Average, mg	Range, mg
External iron loss	170	150–200
Expansion of red-blood-cell mass	450	200–600
Fetal iron	270	200–370
Iron in placenta and cord	90	30–170
Blood loss at delivery	150	90–310
Total requirement[a]	980	580–1,340
Cost of pregnancy[b]	680	440–1,050

[a] Blood loss at delivery not included.
[b] Expansion of red-blood-cell mass not included.
SOURCE: After Council on Foods and Nutrition, 1968. Courtesy of the *Journal of the American Medical Association*.

the daily requirement, as Table 1 indicates. Since the average American diet provides about 6 mg of iron per thousand kcal (Monsen *et al.*, 1967), iron intake from dietary sources is borderline for teenage girls and women and may be inadequate for infants and pregnant women (AMA Council on Foods and Nutrition, 1968: Committee on Dietary Allowances, 1974). Nevertheless, a woman who has sufficient iron stores to provide for increase in hemoglobin mass during pregnancy and who breast feeds her infant for 6 months (thereby delaying the return of menstruation) will have her iron needs covered by an adequate intake of dietary iron (FAO/WHO Expert Group, 1970).

The diagnostic features of iron deficiency are summarized in Table 1. To this should be added the fact that 5 mg or less of iron/100 g of liver tissue is indicative of depletion of the storage pool to the extent that iron-deficiency anemia may be either present or anticipated with any further depletion (Sturgeon and Shoden, 1971).

As stated in footnote *b* to Table 1, the amount of iron required to meet the needs of pregnancy should usually be met by iron supplementation in the latter half of pregnancy, since it cannot usually be derived from diet. The Committee on Maternal Nutrition (1970) recommends supplementation with 30–60 mg of iron daily (i.e., 150–300 mg of ferrous sulfate) during pregnancy. The physician should use his judgment in this regard, based on knowledge of the patient, the dietary habits, the fact that iron deficiency is frequent in pregnant women, and his evaluation of the blood and iron status of the particular patient (Herbert, 1975a). He may routinely give iron (Wallerstein, 1973).

In general, oral ferrous sulfate, the least expensive iron preparation, is the drug of choice for treating iron deficiency. A detailed discussion of iron therapy is presented elsewhere (Herbert, 1972; Herbert, 1975a). It is important to remember that the duration of oral therapy for iron deficiency should be approximately 6 months, since a lesser duration will not adequately replete body iron stores. The physician must remember that the iron deficiency may have developed in association with menorrhagia; if that menorrhagia persists, iron therapy may have to persist as well so that the iron loss in blood does not again produce a negative iron balance.

About 3–4 percent of the iron in vegetable foods and 15–20 percent of the iron in animal foods is absorbed. Heme iron accounts for about one-third the iron in animal tissues, but the heme in a moderate portion of meat, fish, or poultry may supply up to one-third of the daily requirement because it is 5 to 10 times as absorbable as inorganic iron in food (Cook, 1978). Nonheme iron absorption is *enhanced* by vitamin C and a ''meat tissue factor'' (not found in milk, eggs, or cheese); it is *inhibited* by eggs, bran, tea, EDTA, and calcium phosphate (Cook, 1978). Thus, the amount of iron absorbed from a particular meal is dependent largely on its proportion of heme and nonheme iron, and its content of ascorbic acid and animal food, and iron deficiency, is much more frequent in vegetarians.

The high frequency of iron deficiency in infants correlates with diets consisting largely of milk, so the maximum incidence is between 6 months and 2 years of age, and it is corrected by eating a mixed diet, so by age 5 it has fallen considerably. The 0.2–0.3 μg Fe/ml breast milk is adequate to the requirements of the exclusively breast-fed infant until birth weight is tripled. When breast feeding is discontinued before age 6 months, the use of formula rather than fresh cow's milk reduces the risk of intestinal blood loss. Cow's milk is higher in iron and lower in lactoferrin than human milk, but the iron in breast milk is better absorbed (Lockhart, 1979).

Bothwell and Charlton note (1973) that use of the traditional iron pot instead of aluminum cookware to prepare their predominantly cereal diet (and traditional drinks) made iron deficiency anemia very infrequent in Bantu women, but made iron overload disease frequent in Bantu men. The striking effect of cooking in an iron skillet on iron content of food is illustrated by them in Table 3.

FOLATE-DEFICIENCY ANEMIA

Studies carried out under the aegis of the World Health Organization (1968) and by Baker and DeMaeyer (1979) in various countries suggest that up to a third of all the pregnant women in the world have folate deficiency. In a recent study in a New York City municipal clinic, our group (Herbert *et al.*, 1975) found tissue deficiency of folic acid, as measured by a red-cell folate

TABLE 3 Effect of Cooking in Iron Skillet (Dutch Oven) on Fe Content of Foods

Food	Cooling Time, min	Iron Content, mg/100 gm Glass Dish	Iron Content, mg/100 gm Dutch Oven
Spaghetti sauce	180	3.0	87.5
Gravy	20	0.43	5.9
Potatoes, fried	30	0.45	3.8
Rice casserole	45	1.4	5.2
Beef hash	45	1.52	5.2
Apple butter	120	0.47	52.5
Scrambled eggs	3	1.7	4.1

SOURCE: Bothwell and Charlton, 1973.

level below 150 ng/ml, present in 16 percent of 110 sequential pregnant women at the time of their first prenatal visit to the clinic. A further 14 percent had red-cell folate levels in the range "suggestive but not conclusive for tissue folate depletion" (150–199 ng/ml). It was suggested that daily ingestion of one fresh or fresh-frozen uncooked fruit or vegetable or fruit juice could have prevented this folate deficiency.

These studies add to a growing body of evidence that nutritional deficiency of folic acid is prevalent among Americans of poor economic status. Based on findings up until 1970, Pritchard, writing for the Committee on Maternal Nutrition of the Food and Nutrition Board (1970), recommended that folic acid supplements should be taken throughout pregnancy. Subsequently, the data of the Ten-State Nutrition Survey (1968–70) became available. Although that survey found that "the mean serum folate values were, with few exceptions, above the acceptable level of 6 ng/ml and the mean red cell folate values were in the acceptable range of 150–650 ng/ml," a more detailed evaluation indicates a real problem in fact exists, obscured by the use of mean values alone (Herbert *et al.*, 1975). The mean values obscured the existence of substantial numbers of actual values sufficiently below the mean as to suggest widespread folic acid deficiency. This is indicated by the data from the Survey Director for Massachusetts of the Ten-State Nutrition Survey (Edozien, 1972).

In Massachusetts, serum and red-cell folates were measured on most of the samples collected. Of all the 1,087 Massachusetts blood samples from females on which such estimations were made, 25.6 percent had red-cell folate values below 150 ng/ml. This includes 115 pregnant women, all of whom were receiving prenatal clinic care, in the economically poor

Roxbury–Dorchester area, and most of whom were receiving vitamin supplements, presumably containing folic acid. Among these pregnant women, 7.1 percent had red-cell folate values below 160 ng/ml and 7.1 percent had serum folate levels below 3 ng/ml. It is probably relevant that the over 10,000 individuals surveyed in Massachusetts were randomly selected from enumeration districts with the lowest average income (lowest quartile) according to the 1960 census (Ten-State Survey, 1968–70), and poverty and folate deficiency tend to run hand in hand (Herbert, 1968; Kahn *et al.*, 1970). As the Massachusetts report noted (Edozien, 1972), "The results suggest that the diets currently eaten by a large segment of the population cannot provide the allowance of folic acid recommended for optimal health and, therefore, that dietary deficiency of folic acid may pose a major nutritional problem. Considered together with the finding of a high prevalence of low plasma vitamin A levels, it would appear that these diets contain insufficient amounts of green leafy vegetables which are major sources of both folic acid and provitamin A. Current processes for preservation, storage and preparation of foods may also destroy a high proportion of the folate in foods."

The hazard to mother and fetus of folate deficiency in the absence of frank anemia is unclear and has been extensively reviewed (Rothman, 1970). Studies from South Africa suggest that folate supplements in this situation decrease the incidence of prematurity (Baumslag *et al.*, 1970) and cause significant elevation of hemoglobin levels (Colman *et al.*, 1975 a, b, c), suggesting that even mild deficiency may limit DNA synthesis. Prospective studies of the effects on the fetus are difficult to interpret because folate administration invariably starts only after the period of maximum fetal susceptibility in the first trimester. However, animal experiments demonstrate a consistent teratogenic effect of folate deprivation from the time of conception, dependent on the duration of the experiment (Herbert *et al.*, 1975).

Thus, in the light of present knowledge it appears appropriate to correct folate deficiency in pregnancy. The implementation of this principle by improving the quality and quantity of available food is a long-term ideal limited by custom and economic circumstances. For this reason, the Joint FAO/WHO Expert Committee on Nutrition has recommended that food fortification should be considered as an immediate possibility for the improvement of intake of any deficient nutrient (FAO/WHO Expert Committee, 1971). A series of studies indicate that fortification of staple foods with folic aicd is feasible, safe, effective, and in accordance with the recommendations of the Expert Committee (Colman *et al.*, 1974a,b,c, 1975a,b,c). With adequate fortification, possible hazards of folate deficiency in early pregnancy would be averted. Until such fortification is practiced, administration of folic acid tablets, 200–400 μg/day, is appropriate for all pregnant women, with 300 μg probably adequate for any pregnant population group (Herbert, 1977).

The evidence relating folate deficiency in pregnancy to presence in the offspring of mental retardation and other defects in central nervous system function and development is reviewed elsewhere (Herbert and Tisman, 1973). This evidence is, as yet, far from conclusive but does constitute one more slight increment in the balance favoring the concept of daily folate supplementation throughout pregnancy.

In 1975, there was a National Academy of Sciences "Workshop on Human Folate Requirements," whose proceedings were published in 1977. That workshop included papers presenting the latest information on distribution of folates in food, food folate availability, results of several surveys to detect folate deficiency in certain American population groups, and reviews of the folic acid requirement in children, adults, and in situations of increased need. To briefly summarize the findings most pertinent to nutritional anemias: Measurement of serum and red-cell folate together constitute the best method for delineating the existence of folate deficiency; food folate availability is affected by various constituents present in different foodstuffs; pregnancy increases folate requirement.

The minimal daily adult requirement for folic acid, which must be absorbed from food to sustain normality, is in the range of 50 μg daily (Herbert, 1968), and the Food and Nutrition Board (1974) recommends that the diets of adults contain 400 μg daily. This requirement appears to be approximately doubled by pregnancy. Thus, if a woman is absorbing from her food in the range of 100 μg of folic acid daily from the start of pregnancy, she may not need supplementation, but assuming lesser stores than normal at the start of pregnancy, 200–300 μg of folate supplementation daily may be necessary (Herbert, 1975; Herbert, 1977). The Food and Nutrition Board (1974) recommends a daily dietary intake of 800 μg during pregnancy and 600 μg during lactation.

Although serum and red-cell folate may be lowered by the use of oral contraceptives (Smith *et al.*, 1975; Prasad *et al.*, 1975), it is not yet clear that folate supplementation is needed by women taking such products (Anonymous, 1973; Lindenbaum, 1975). This folate need would probably be adequately met by one fresh uncooked vegetable, fruit, or fruit juice daily (Herbert, 1975b).

VITAMIN B_{12}

Although serum vitamin B_{12} level falls in pregnancy (Cooper, 1973) and may also fall with the use of oral contraceptives (Wertalik *et al.*, 1972; Smith *et al.*, 1975), tissue levels of vitamin B_{12} may remain normal and vitamin B_{12}

deficiency anemia has not seemed to be a problem (Wertalik *et al.*, 1972). From evidence so far, vitamin B_{12} deficiency anemia is rarely a dietary problem in the United States (Herbert, 1975b). In population groups where vitamin B_{12} deficiency is common due to vegetarianism, such vitamin B_{12} deficiency would be increased by the metabolic stress in pregnancy, including the fetal drain on maternal stores of about 0.3 μg B_{12}/day (Herbert, 1968; WHO, 1970) and by a mean of 0.3 μg B_{12}/day lost in breast milk during lactation (WHO, 1970). It is for these reasons that the recommended dietary allowance (Food and Nutrition Board, 1974) for vitamin B_{12} was raised from the 3 μg for adults in general to 4 μg for pregnant or lactating females.

Certain microorganisms and all animal protein are the sole source of dietary vitamin B_{12}. Thus, any diet devoid of animal protein, or not containing microorganisms that synthesize the vitamin, will eventually produce vitamin B_{12} deficiency, unless the diet is supplemented with the vitamin. Certain seaweeds and legume nodules contain microorganisms that synthesize the vitamin; eating these foods and unwashed food contaminated with fecal microorganisms that synthesize the vitamin delays the onset of vitamin B_{12} deficiency.

REFERENCES

AMA Council on Foods and Nutrition. 1968. Iron deficiency in the United States. JAMA 203:407–412.

AMA Council on Foods and Nutrition. 1972. Iron in enriched wheat flour, farina, bread, buns and rolls. JAMA 220:855–859.

Anonymous. 1973. Feminins and other vitamin–mineral supplements for women taking oral contraceptives. Med. Lett. 15:81–82.

Anonymous. 1974. Topical and systematic contraceptive agents. Med. Lett. 16:37–40.

Anonymous. 1975. Cu-7, a copper containing IUD. Med. Lett. 17:26–27.

Baker, S. J., and E. M. DeMaeyer. 1979. Nutritional anemia: Its understanding and control with special reference to the work of the World Health Organization. Am. J. Clin. Nutr. 32:368–417.

Baumslag, N., T. Edelstein, and J. Metz. 1970. Reduction of incidence of prematurity by folic acid supplementation in pregnancy. Br. Med. J. 1:16–17.

Bothwell, T. H., and R. W. Charlton. 1973. Iron deficiency geographically speaking. *In* W. H. Crosby, ed. Iron. Medcom, New York.

Colman, N., M. Barker, R. Green, and J. Metz. 1974a. Prevention of folate deficiency in pregnancy by food fortification. Am. J. Clin. Nutr. 27:339.

Colman, N., J. V. Larsen, M. Barker, E. A. Barker, R. Green, and J. Metz. 1974b. Prevention of folate deficiency by food fortification. V. A pilot field trial of folic acid-fortified maize meal. S. Afr. Med. J. 48:1763.

Colman, N., R. Green, K. Stevens, and J. Metz. 1974c. Prevention of folate deficiency by food fortification. VI. The antimegaloblastic effect of folic acid-fortified maize meal. S. Afr. Med. J. 48:1795.

Colman, N., R. Green, and J. Metz. 1975a. Prevention of folate deficiency by food fortification. II. Absorption of folic acid from fortified staple foods. Am. J. Clin. Nutr. 28:459–464.

Colman, N., J. V. Larsen, M. Barker, E. A. Barker, R. Green, and J. Metz, 1975b. Prevention of folate deficiency by food fortification. III. Effect in pregnant subjects of varying amounts of added folic acid. Am. J. Clin. Nutr. 28:465–470.

Colman, N., E. A. Barker, M. Barker, R. Green, and J. Metz. 1975c. Prevention of folate deficiency by food fortification. IV. Identification of target groups in addition to pregnant women in an adult rural population. Am. J. Clin. Nutr. 28:471–476.

Cook, J. D. 1978. Food iron availability. Food Nutr. News 49(3):1,4. (National Live Stock and Meat Board, Chicago)

Cooper, B. 1973. Folate and vitamin B_{12} in pregnancy. Clin. Haemat. 2:461–476.

Committee on Dietary Allowances. 1974. Recommended dietary allowances. Food and Nutrition Board, National Research Council, National Academy of Sciences, Washington, D.C.

Committee on Maternal Nutrition. 1970. Maternal nutrition and the course of pregnancy. Food and Nutrition Board, National Research Council, National Academy of Sciences, Washington, D.C.

Dorland's illustrated medical dictionary, 25th ed. 1974. W. B. Saunders, Philadelphia.

Edozien, J. C. 1972. National Nutrition Survey, Massachusetts, July 1969–June 1971. Report of the Survey Director to the Commissioner for Public Health, Commonwealth of Massachusetts, Boston. (Kindly supplied to us by Derek Robinson, M.D., Director, Division of Community Operations, Department of Public Health, Commonwealth of Massachusetts.)

Fairbanks, V. F., J. L. Fahey, and E. Beutler, eds. 1971. Clinical disorders of iron metabolism, 2d ed. Grune and Stratton, New York and London.

FAO/WHO Expert Committee on Nutrition. 1971. Food fortification. WHO Tech. Rep. Ser. No. 477.

FAO/WHO Expert Group. 1970. Requirements of ascorbic acid, vitamin D, vitamin B_{12}, folate and iron. WHO Tech. Rep. Ser. No. 452. (Purchasable for $1.25 from WHO in Geneva or American Public Health Association, 1740 Broadway, New York, NY 10019. Available in English, French, Spanish, Russian, and Chinese.)

Food and Nutrition Board, National Research Council. 1977. Folic acid: Biochemistry and physiology in relation to the human nutrition requirement. National Academy of Sciences, Washington, D.C.

Hallberg, L., A.-M. Hogdahl, L. Nilsson, and G. Rybo. 1966. Menstrual blood loss, a population study: Variation at different ages and attempts to define normality.

Herbert, V. 1968. Nutritional requirements of vitamin B_{12} and folic acid. Am. J. Clin. Nutr. 21:743–752.

Herbert, V. 1970. Introduction to the nutritional anemias. Semin. Haemat. 7:2–5.

Herbert, V. 1972. Oral iron therapy. *In* W. H. Crosby, ed. Iron. Medcom, New York.

Herbert, V. 1975a. Drugs effective in iron-deficiency and other hypochromic anemias. Pages 1309–1323 *in* L. S. Goodman and A. Gilman, eds. The pharmacological basis of therapeutics, 5th ed. Macmillan, New York.

Herbert, V. 1975b. Drugs effective in megaloblastic anemias. Vitamin B_{12} and folic acid. Pages 1324–1349 *in* L. S. Goodman and A. Gilman, eds. The pharmacological basis of therapeutics, 5th ed. Macmillan, New York.

Herbert, V. 1977. Folic acid requirements in adults (including pregnant and lactating females). *In* Folic acid. Food and Nutrition Board, National Academy of Sciences, Washington, D.C.

Herbert, V., and G. Tisman. 1973. Effects of deficiencies of folic acid and vitamin B_{12} on central nervous system function and development. Pages 373–392 *in* G. Gaull, ed. Biology of brain dysfunction, vol. 1. Plenum Press, New York and London.

Herbert, V., N. Colman, M. Spivack, E. Ocasio, V. Ghanta, K. Kimmel, L. Brenner, J. Freundlich, and J. Scott. 1975. Folic acid deficiency in the United States: Folate assays in a prenatal clinic. Am. J. Obstet. Gynecol. 123:175–179.

Kahn, S. B., S. Fein, S. Rigberg, and I. Brodsky. 1970. Correlation of folate metabolism and socioeconomic status in pregnancy and in patients taking oral contraceptives. Am. J. Obstet. Gynecol. 108:931–935.

Layrisse, M. 1975. Iron nutriture. Pages 148–154 *in* P. L. White and N. Selvey, eds. Proceedings, Western Hemisphere Nutrition Congress IV. Publishing Sciences Group, Acton, Mass.

Lindenbaum, J., N. Whitehead, and F. Reyner. 1975. Oral contraceptive hormones, folate metabolism, and the cervical epithelium. Am. J. Clin. Nutr. 28:346–353.

Lockhart, J. D. 1979. Breast milk. Contemp. Nutr. 4(1):1–2 (General Mills, Minneapolis).

Monsen, E. R., I. N. Kuhn, and C. A. Finch. 1967. Iron status of menstruating women. Am. J. Clin. Nutr. 20:842–849.

Moore, C. V., and R. Dubach. 1956. Metabolism and requirements of iron in the human. JAMA 162:197–204.

Prasad, A. S., K. Y. Lei, D. Oberleas, K. S. Moghissi, and J. C. Stryker. 1975. Effect of oral contraceptive agents on nutrients. II. Vitamins. Am. J. Clin. Nutr. 28:385–391.

Rothman, D. 1970. Folic acid in pregnancy. Am. J. Obstet. Gynecol. 108:149–175.

Rybo, G. 1970. Menstrual loss of iron. Pages 163–171 *in* L. Hallberg, H.-G. Harwerth, and A. Vannotti, eds. Iron deficiency. Academic Press, London and New York.

Scott, D. E., and J. A. Pritchard, 1967. Iron deficiency in healthy young college women. JAMA 199:897–900.

Scott, D. E., J. A. Pritchard, A. S. Saltin, and J. M. Humphreys. 1970. Iron deficiency during pregnancy. Pages 491–503 *in* L. Hallberg, H.-G. Harwerth, and A. Vannotti, eds. Iron deficiency, Academic Press, London and New York.

Smith, J. L., G. A. Goldsmith, and J. D. Lawrence. 1975. Effects of oral contraceptive steroids on vitamin and lipid levels in serum. Am. J. Clin. Nutr. 28:377–384.

Sturgeon, P., and A. Shoden. 1971. Total liver storage iron in normal populations of the U.S.A. Am. J. Clin. Nutr. 24:469–474.

Symposium. 1975. Effects of oral contraceptive hormones on nutrient metabolism. Am. J. Clin. Nutr. 28:333–402, 521–560.

Ten-State Nutrition Survey. 1968–70. U.S. Department of Health, Education, and Welfare, Center for Disease Control, Atlanta, Ga. DHEW Publ. No. (HSM) 72-8130 through 8134.

Wallerstein, R. O. 1973. Iron metabolism and iron deficiency during pregnancy. Clin. Haemat. 2:453–460.

Wertalik, L. F., E. N. Metz, A. F. LoBuglio, and S. P. Balcerzak. 1972. Decreased serum B_{12} levels with oral contraceptive use. JAMA 221:1371–1374.

WHO Scientific Group. 1968. Nutritional anaemias. WHO Tech. Rep. Ser. No. 405. (Purchasable for $1.00 from Publication Distribution and Sales, World Health Organization, 1211 Geneva 27, Switzerland.)

Wintrobe, M. M. 1973. The proposed increase in the iron fortification of wheat products. Nutr. Today 8:18–20.

APPENDIX D Participants and Observers

Workshop on Methods for the Collection of Aggregate Data on Food Consumption

OCTOBER 18–19, 1978

PARTICIPANTS

I. J. ABRAMS, Market Research Corporation of America, Chicago, Ill.
ROBERT W. ALSTRIN, Food Service Marketing, Armour Food Company, Phoenix, Ariz.
WILLIAM ASH, Group Marketing Research, Durkee Foods Division, SCM Corporation, Cleveland, Ohio
CHARLES J. BATES, American Maize Products, Co., Hammond, Ind.
HAROLD F. BREIMYER, Department of Agricultural Economics, University of Missouri—Columbia, Columbia, Mich.
MAHLON A. BURNETTE, Grocery Manufacturers of America, Inc., Washington, D.C.
OLIVER CASTLE, A. C. Nielsen Company, Northbrook, Ill.
ALLAN L. FORBES, Nutrition and Consumer Sciences, Food and Drug Administration, Washington, D.C.
WILLIAM GAHR, Food Group, U.S. General Accounting Office, Washington, D.C.
THOMAS B. GRIMSHAW, Selling Areas Marketing, Inc., New York, N.Y.
HELEN A. GUTHRIE, Nutrition Program, Pennsylvania State University, University Park.
TIMOTHY A. HAMMONDS, Food Marketing Institute, Washington, D.C.
HAROLD B. HOUSER, Department of Biometry, Case Western Reserve University, Cleveland, Ohio
GENE HUDAK Technomic Research Associates, Chicago, Ill.
HARRY L. JACOBS, Behavioral Sciences Division, Food Sciences Laboratory, Natick Research and Development Command, Natick, Mass.
ALDEN MANCHESTER, Economics, Statistics, and Cooperative Service, U.S. Department of Agriculture, Washington, D.C.
ROBERT O. NESHEIM, Science and Technology, The Quaker Oats Company, Chicago, Ill.
MARY O'BRIEN, Committee on Science and Technology, U.S. Congress, Washington, D.C.
ROBERT PEARL, Silver Spring, Md.
MILO SUNDERHAUF, Office of Federal Statistical Policy and Analysis, U.S. Department of Commerce, Washington, D.C.

LAWRENCE VAN MEIR, Economics and Statistics Division, National Food Processors Association, Washington, D.C.

JOHN E. VANDERVEEN, Division of Nutrition, Food and Drug Administration, Washington, D.C.

Workshop on Evaluation of Methods for Obtaining Food Consumption Data

NOVEMBER 8–10, 1978

PARTICIPANTS

I. J. ABRAMS, Market Research Corporation of America, Chicago, Ill.
VIRGINIA A. BEAL, Department of Food Science and Nutrition, University of Massachusetts, Amherst, Mass.
MARGUERITE C. BURK, International Studies in Human Ecology, Howard University, Washington, D.C.
DORIS H. CALLOWAY, Department of Nutritional Sciences, University of California, Berkeley, Calif.
CLAIRE M. CASSIDY, University of Maryland, College Park.
MARY DOUGLAS, Research on Culture, Russell Sage Foundation, New York, N.Y.
WILLIAM GAHR, Food Group, U.S. General Accounting Office, Washington, D.C.
SAMUEL GREENHOUSE, Department of Statistics, George Washington University, Washington, D.C.
HELEN A. GUTHRIE, Nutrition Program, Pennsylvania State University, University Park
GAIL G. HARRISON, Department of Family and Community Medicine, College of Medicine, University of Arizona, Tucson, Ariz.
HAROLD B. HOUSER, Department of Biometry, Case Western Reserve University, Cleveland, Ohio
OGDEN C. JOHNSON, Scientific Affairs, Hershey Foods Corporation, Hershey, Pa.
J. PATRICK MADDEN, Agricultural Economics, Pennsylvania State University, University Park.
ROBERT O. NESHEIM, Science and Technology, The Quaker Oats Company, Chicago, Ill.
ROBERT PEARL, Silver Spring, Md.
DIVA SANJUR, Division of Nutritional Science, Cornell University, Ithaca, N.Y.
DAVID D. SCHNAKENBERG, Bioenergetics Division, Letterman Army Institute of Research, Presidio of San Francisco, Calif.
HOWARD G. SCHUTZ, Center for Consumer Research, University of California—Davis, Davis, Calif.
CHARLOTTE M. YOUNG, Minneapolis, Minn.

OBSERVERS

CHARLES J. BATES, American Maize Products Co., Hammond, Ind.

KATHERINE CLANCY, Division of National Advertising, Federal Trade Commission, Washington, D.C.

CONNIE MARIE DRESSER, Division of Health Examination Statistics, National Center for Health Statistics, Hyattsville, Md.

STEPHEN J. HIEMSTRA, Economic Analysis and Program Evaluation Staff, U.S. Department of Agriculture, Washington, D.C.

HAROLD NISSELSON, Statistical Standards and Methodology, Bureau of Census, Washington, D.C.

ELEANOR PAO, Food Consumption Research Group, Consumer and Food Economics Institute, U.S. Department of Agriculture, Hyattsville, Md.

RAYMOND E. SCHUCKER, Bureau of Foods, Food and Drug Administration, Washington, D.C.

RAYMOND C. STOKES, Division of Consumer Studies, Food and Drug Administration, Washington, D.C.

MILO B. SUNDERHAUF, Office of Federal Statistical Policy and Analysis, U.S. Department of Commerce, Washington, D.C.

JOHN E. VANDERVEEN, Division of Nutrition, Food and Drug Administration, Washington, D.C.

MARY MARGARET WILSON, Nutrition Statistics Branch, Division of Health Examination Statistics, National Center for Health Statistics, Hyattsville, Md.

Workshop on Nutrition and Health Status Indicators

MARCH 21–23, 1979

PARTICIPANTS

I. J. ABRAMS, Menu Census Services, Market Research Corporation of America, Chicago, Ill.
BASIL G. BIBBY, Department of Caries Research, Eastman Dental Center, Rochester, N.Y.
DORIS H. CALLOWAY, Department of Nutritional Sciences, University of California—Berkeley, Berkeley, Calif.
GAIL G. HARRISON, Department of Family and Community Medicine, College of Medicine, University of Arizona, Tucson, Ariz.
VICTOR M. HAWTHORNE, Department of Epidemiology, School of Public Health, University of Michigan, Ann Arbor, Mich.
D. MARK HEGSTED, Human Nutrition Center, U.S. Department of Agriculture, Washington, D.C.
VICTOR HERBERT, SUNY Downstate Medical Center and Hematology and Nutrition Laboratory, VA Hospital, Bronx, New York.
HAROLD B. HOUSER, Department of Biometry, Case Western Reserve University, Cleveland, Ohio
FRANCIS E. JOHNSTON, Department of Anthropology, University of Pennsylvania, Philadelphia.
JEAN A. T. PENNINGTON, Biology Department, City College of San Francisco, San Francisco, Calif.
ROBERT O. NESHEIM, Science and Technology, The Quaker Oats Company, Chicago, Ill.
DWAYNE M. REED, Epidemiological Studies, Department of Health Services, Berkeley, Calif.
ARNOLD E. SCHAEFFER, Swanson Center for Nutrition, Inc., Omaha, Nebr.
HOWARD G. SCHUTZ, Center for Consumer Research, University of California—Davis, Davis, Calif.

OBSERVERS

SIDNEY ABRAHAM, Nutrition Statistics Bureau, National Center for Health Statisitics, Hyattsville, Md.

ALLAN L. FORBES, Nutrition and Consumer Sciences, Food and Drug Administration, Washington, D.C.

JAMES W. HICKS, Nutrition Division, Bureau of Smallpox Eradication, Center for Disease Control, Atlanta, Ga.

GRACE OSTENSO, House Committee on Science and Technology, U.S. Congress, Washington, D.C.

JOHN E. VANDERVEEN, Division of Nutrition, Food and Drug Administration, Washington, D.C.

KATHERINE CLANCY, Division of National Advertising, Federal Trade Commission, Washington, D.C.

ROBERT C. DOSTER, Basic Research, Carnation Research Laboratories, Van Nuys, Calif.